Imaging the Acutely Ill Patient: A Clinician's Guide

W0091860

Commissioning Editor: Sue Hodgson
Project Development Manager: Paul Fam
Project Manager: Scott Millar
Designer: Jayne Jones

Imaging the Acutely Ill Patient: A Clinician's Guide

Barry E. Kelly MD FRCS (Ed) FRCR FFRRCSI

Consultant Radiologist, The Royal Victoria Hospital, Belfast
and
Honorary Lecturer in Radiology, The Queen's University, Belfast

Colin S. McArdle
MD FRCS(Eng), FRCS(Glas), FRCS(Edin)

Professor of Surgery, University Department of Surgery
Edinburgh Royal Infirmary, Edinburgh

 W. B. SAUNDERS COMPANY LTD

London · Philadelphia · Toronto · Sydney · Tokyo

WB SAUNDERS
An imprint of Harcourt Publishers Limited

© Harcourt Publishers Limited 2001

 is a registered trademark of Harcourt Publishers Limited

The right of Barry E. Kelly and Colin S. McArdle to be identified as authors of this work has been asserted by them in accordance with the Copyright, Designs and Patents Act 1988

First published 2001

ISBN 0-7020-2434-1

British Library Cataloguing in Publication Data
A catalogue record for this book is available from the British Library

Library of Congress Cataloging in Publication Data
A catalog record for this book is available from the Library of Congress

Note
Medical knowledge is constantly changing. As new information becomes available, changes in treatment, procedures, equipment and the use of drugs become necessary. The editors/authors/contributors and the publishers have, as far as it is possible, taken care to ensure that the information given in this text is accurate and up to date. However, readers are strongly advised to confirm that the information, especially with regard to drug usage, complies with the latest legislation and standards of practice.

The
publisher's
policy is to use
**paper manufactured
from sustainable forests**

Printed in China

www.harcourt-international.com

Bringing you products from all Harcourt Health Sciences companies including Baillière Tindall, Churchill Livingstone, Mosby and W.B. Saunders

- ▶ **Browse** for latest information on new books, journals and electronic products

- ▶ **Search** for information on over 20 000 published titles with full product information including tables of contents and sample chapters

- ▶ **Keep up to date** with our extensive publishing programme in your field by registering with eAlert or requesting postal updates

- ▶ **Secure online ordering** with prompt delivery, as well as full contact details to order by phone, fax or post

- ▶ **News** of special features and promotions

If you are based in the following countries, please visit the country-specific site to receive full details of product availability and local ordering information

USA: www.harcourthealth.com

Canada: www.harcourtcanada.com

Australia: www.harcourt.com.au

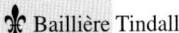 Baillière Tindall   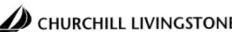 CHURCHILL LIVINGSTONE   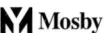 Mosby   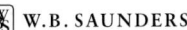 W.B. SAUNDERS

Contents

Preface

I wrote this book with one person in mind: me. Years ago, as a pre-Fellowship surgical trainee, many lonely on-call nights were spent peering intently at viewing boxes in casualty, the ward and the operating theatre. I marvelled at those little pieces of celluloid. I knew that they must contain oceans of information, but the bulk of this knowledge was, for me, unattainable.

There were of course, many fine imaging texts available for the non-radiologist. It seemed to me, however, that these tended to concentrate on CT, ultrasound, nuclear medicine and contrast examinations. I needed something more elementary; a scheme for interpreting plain films that was accessible to the non-radiologist without being over simplistic.

Years later, and with the help of many understanding and patient tutors, I began to understand how to demystify those enigmatic radiographs. This is what I have set out to do in this short work.

With my co-author, Professor Colin McArdle, we have attempted to pare the body systems down to their radiological basics, and guide the novice through a systematic system for analysing the plain radiograph.

Throughout this book, plain radiographs have been our focus. I always did, and still do find these the most challenging of films. They also still represent, for most of the world's health systems, *the gatekeeper*. Progression to more complex imaging may well depend on the correct deduction being made from the plain radiograph.

We have not, however, confined ourselves to plain films; ultrasound, CT, MRI, colour Doppler, and angiograms are all represented. These hopefully have been used to emphasise a diagnosis or make a point.

I hope that this book helps your decision making on lonely on-call nights. Those of us who were that soldier, salute you.

Barry Kelly
Belfast.
October 2000

"For every mistake resulting from lack of knowledge, ten occur from lack of looking."

JA Lindsay
1923

Foreword

It is a pleasure and an honour to write a foreword to this intriguing textbook. The principal author modestly claims that the idea of the book was to help surgeons in training understand a bit about the 'pieces of celluloid' which they have to interpret in the middle of the night. Even though times are changing and the pieces of celluloid are being replaced by computer based images, the principle remains sound: a good surgeon should still be able to understand the rudiments of radiology in order to balance the strength of the radiological evidence with the clinical symptoms and signs.

The book is very much a personal glimpse of the authors' collective experience and, because the work comes from two busy teaching hospitals, this is extensive. The book contains a wealth of useful information for many groups of medical and para-medical personnel. Indeed trainee radiologists in the first few years of training would find much of value here, as did a middle-aged consultant!

The book is easy to read with excellent labelled images and illustrative line diagrams. Each chapter can be covered in about an hour. This short book cannot be comprehensive but this is part of its charm. Indeed the chapter titles themselves and the contents illustrate the areas where confusion is likely and guidance is needed. Thus chest imaging warrants about twentyfive per cent of the book, the acute abdomen nearly 20%, hepatobiliary disease 10%, urological problems 20%, etc. This is a fair reflection of what comes through the door as acute admissions in a general hospital.

Writing radiological text-books is no easy matter. The technology changes so fast that gospel one day is history the next. The authors have done well in retaining some of the tried and tested investigations such as the intravenous urogram. Even though there is increasing use of spiral computed tomography for renal colic, this is not yet universal and, in any case, the principles gleaned from decades of IVU experience will still apply in full. The good news is that the rapid advances occurring in radiology will necessitate another edition of the book in a few years time. Given the obvious enthusiasm of the authors this will also be a very good read!

I congratulate the authors on producing this useful book, which more than fulfils the stated mission. Many health care workers will be able to handle the acutely ill patient with much more confidence after assimilating the information contained within. I wish the authors and the book well.

Adrian K Dixon
Professor of Radiology
Addenbrooke's NHS Trust and
the University of Cambridge

Acknowledgements

Although this is a short work, many have generously given of their time and expertise. Colin McArdle, my former surgical mentor and co-author, was instrumental in every stage of this project. His unfailing eye for detail, logical approach and wealth of clinical experience was indispensable. His constant good humour, often in the face of severe provocation from his co-author, was sincerely appreciated.

I would like to express my sincere gratitude to my interventional colleague, Dr Peter Ellis, for co-authoring the chapter on vascular imaging, to all my colleagues who read the evolving drafts and provided very helpful criticism; and also those who contributed images: Drs Chris Boyd, Miriam Buckley, Annie Paterson, and Paul Rice.

I would also wish to acknowledge the significant influence of Dr Edwin McIlrath, emeritus Head of Department of Radiology, Royal Victoria Hospital, for demonstrating how to bridge the gap between the clinical specialities and radiology so effectively that one couldn't see the join.

Thanks also to all those at WB Saunders, particularly Sue Hodgson, Paul Fam and Scott Millar for steering me gently in the right direction.

Finally, and most importantly to Susan, Katie and Rosie for unceasing support and understanding.

BK

1 | Principles of Radiology

Topics included in this chapter

- Conventional Radiography
- Conventional Tomography
- Ultrasound
- Doppler Imaging
- Computed Axial Tomography
- Magnetic Resonance Imaging
- Radiation Dose from Diagnostic Imaging

CONVENTIONAL RADIOGRAPHY

X-rays form part of the electromagnetic spectrum and are produced in an evacuated x-ray tube. A tungsten cathode filament inside the tube is heated to over 2000°C. This liberates electrons which are focused on to a tungsten anode by applying a very large potential difference (50–150 kV) between the anode and the cathode. Most of the radiation produced is absorbed by the tube casing, but a small amount escapes through a window in the casing. This resultant beam of radiation is able to pass through the human body and be detected by a photographic film.

Photographic effect

Within a film cassette, the photographic film lies between two fluorescent screens.

When exposed to an x-ray beam, light emitted from these screens causes blackening of the film's emulsion after it has been developed.

Radiographic appearances

Tissues can be differentiated because of their differential absorption of the x-ray beam. Air produces the least absorption, and therefore the most film blackening. Soft tissues (except fat) all absorb the same amount of the x-ray beam, and therefore are of the same shade of grey. Fat, which absorbs slightly less radiation than the other soft tissues, is a shade darker than the others. Calcified structures absorb most and therefore appear white.

1

CONVENTIONAL TOMOGRAPHY

Tomography allows a selected body plane to remain in focus, while blurring out tissues above and below the prechosen level. This is achieved by moving the cassette and the x-ray tube about an axis at the required depth. The tomographic thickness is typically between 1 mm and 1 cm. Tomographic cuts are most commonly used in the intravenous urogram.

ULTRASOUND

The principle of ultrasound scanning is to pass high-frequency sound waves into body tissues and to detect the subsequent returning waves reflected back by internal structures. Sound waves are an energy form that requires a transmission medium. The frequency of ultrasound is greater than 20 000 Hz. Diagnostic ultrasound frequencies range from 1 to 20 MHz. Ultrasound waves are produced in a transducer by using an electromagnetic field to cause an internal arrangement within the architecture of a piezoelectric crystal; this rearrangement alters the crystal's physical shape thus emitting sound waves.

Types of ultrasound

A (amplitude) mode

Echoes are displayed on a cathode ray tube. The height (amplitude) of the trace 'spike' is proportional to the intensity of the echo, and the position of the spike along the horizontal axis indicates the depth in tissue.

B (brightness) mode

A slice of tissue is represented on the screen in the form of dots. These dots are displayed only if they are above a certain intensity.

Grey-scale imaging

The slice of tissue is represented as shades of grey, the shade depending on the echo intensity of the tissue. Although over 64 shades can be differentiated by the scanner, only 10–11 are displayed, as the human eye cannot differentiate more than this.

M (movement) mode

This is used extensively in echocardiography. A continuous trace is produced by the A-mode trace (see above) moving on the screen.

Real-time imaging

Multiple transducer elements are 'arrayed' or combined within the scanhead to produce an instantaneous image. The image can be updated by altering the frame-rate, which typically has a range of between 20 and 200 frames/second. Modern scanners activate the transducer elements electronically in sequence to produce a rectangular image (linear array scanner) or a sector image (phased array scanner).

DOPPLER IMAGING

The Doppler effect describes an alteration of the frequency of sound caused by movement between the observer and the sound source. In Doppler imaging the transducer either emits and receives sound simultaneously using two piezoelectric crystals (continuous wave Doppler), or a single crystal which emits a sound wave and then 'listens' for the returning signal (pulsed wave Doppler). The difference in the returning frequency – the Doppler shift – reflects the speed with which the red blood cells are moving. This can be displayed as a colour image, a spectral trace or an audible signal.

COMPUTED AXIAL TOMOGRAPHY

Computed tomography (CT) produces cross-sectional images using x-rays. These images are acquired typically in the horizontal or 'axial' plane. CT differs from conventional imaging in a number of respects: instead of a photographic film, there are multiple detectors (usually crystal, gas or ceramic); and the x-ray tube rotates around the patient within its gantry. The information derived from the detectors is analysed by a computer using fast Fourier transformations to reconstruct the image. This computer-based reconstruction allows differentiation of many more densities – over 2000 – than can be displayed on conventional x-ray films.

The CT image

The CT image is divided into picture elements, called pixels. The CT number for each pixel represents the average attenuation (or greyness) within a corresponding block of tissue. This block of tissue, or volume element is known as a voxel. The derived attenuation values are given as Hounsfield units; an arbitrary scale. Water density is 0, air approximately -1000 and bone $+1000$ Hounsfield units. Most soft tissues on CT are between -100 and $+100$ Hounsfield units. The range of densities can be manipulated by the operator. The range to be viewed is called the *window width* and the average level the *window centre*.

Spiral (helical) CT

Spiral CT differs from conventional CT in that as the patient moves through the gantry the tube and detectors continue to rotate. Thus a volumetric data set is produced which permits multiplanar reconstruction. The advantage of spiral CT is that the data set produced allows subsequent multiplanar reformatting by the radiologist.

MAGNETIC RESONANCE IMAGING

Magnetic resonance imaging (MRI) produces superb multiplanar images without using ionizing radiation. The physics of MRI are complicated. What follows is very brief summary of the salient points.

3

The nucleus of a hydrogen atom is a single proton. Because it is charged, and it spins, it has magnetic properties. If a strong external magnetic field is applied to hydrogen atoms (like those within human body water), they align themselves either parallel (the vast majority) or antiparallel (the minority) to the external magnetic field. As the majority of the hydrogen atoms are parallel to the external magnetic field, the net magnetic vector will be in the direction of the magnetic field.

The hydrogen atoms, aligned to the external magnetic field, wobble around the field axis with a motion known as *precession*. The frequency of this precession is known as the *Larmor frequency*, and it alters with the magnetic field strength.

If, now, a second magnetic field, known as a radiofrequency (RF) pulse, is applied perpendicular to the first, at the same frequency as the Larmor frequency, extra energy is given to the hydrogen atoms, and their vector alters through 90° to become perpendicular to the original external magnetic field.

Once the RF pulse stops, the acquired extra energy is shed to the surrounding chemical lattice. This is known as the *T1 relaxation*. In addition, the RF pulse will have made the hydrogen atoms spin synchronously. This phenomenon is known as being *in phase*. Once the RF pulse is stopped, the synchronous motion fades, i.e. dephasing occurs. This dephasing is known as the *T2 relaxation*.

The hydrogen atoms (i.e. the patient) are surrounded by magnetic coils. When the RF pulse is applied and the magnetic vector moves through 90°, a current is induced in these surrounding coils. It is this induced current which, following complex computer analysis, allows an image to be produced. The signal strength depends on the proton density and the T1 and T2 relaxation times. *T1 images produce good anatomical detail; T2 images are more sensitive to pathological change in tissue.*

RADIATION DOSE FROM DIAGNOSTIC IMAGING

There is a statutory requirement for all involved in both the requesting and the delivery of radiological examinations to minimize the dose of radiation received by the patient. It is salutary to consider the doses involved in common diagnostic radiological examinations. The examinations performed most commonly are listed below.

It has been calculated that the increased additional lifetime risk of a fatal cancer from a chest x-ray is approximately 1 in 1 000 000. However, the increased risk from an abdominal CT is estimated at 1 in 2000. To put this risk in perspective, the overall risk of a fatal cancer in the adult population is 1 in 3. Nevertheless, as the usage of CT is increasing, and the dose remains static, it is important, when considering the use of this examination, to be aware of the relatively high radiation burden to the patient. The relative doses from commonly requested radiological procedures are given in **Table 1.1**.

Table 1.1 Typical effective doses from diagnostic medical exposures in the 1990s		
Diagnostic procedure	Equivalent number of chest x-rays	Equivalent period of natural background radiation
Limbs and joints	<0.05	<1.5 days
Chest (single PA film)	1	3 days
Skull	3.5	11 days
Thoracic spine	35	4 months
Lumbar spine	65	7 months
Hip	15	7 weeks
Pelvis	35	4 months
Abdomen	50	6 months
IVU	125	14 months
Barium swallow	75	8 months
Barium meal	150	16 months
Barium enema	350	3.2 years
CT brain	115	1 year
CT chest	400	3.6 years
CT abdomen or pelvis	500	4.5 years
Lung ventilation (Xe-133)	15	7 weeks
Lung perfusion (Tc-99m)	50	6 months
Bone scan (Tc-99m)	200	2.7 years
Making the best use of a department of clinical radiology, 4th edn, 1998, Royal College of Radiologists, London		

Further Reading

Armstrong P, Wastie M L 1987 Diagnostic imaging, 2nd edn. Oxford: Blackwell Scientific.

Chapman S, Nakielny R 1986 A guide to radiological procedures, 2nd edn. London: Baillière Tindall.

2 Chest Imaging

EVALUATION OF THE NORMAL CHEST RADIOGRAPH

Technical factors

First, ensure that the technical standard of the anterior chest radiograph is sufficient to be of diagnostic quality. Three particular criteria should be checked: *Rotation*, *Inspiration* and *Penetration* (mnemonic: **RIP**).

Rotation

Check that the medial borders of the clavicle are midway from the spinous process of the projected vertebral body (**Fig. 2.1**). With rotation, the distance between the clavicle and the spinous process opens towards the side of the rotation.

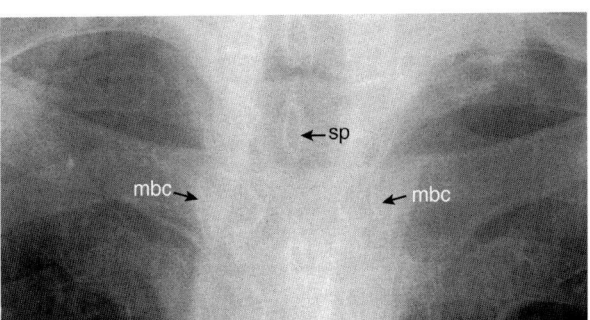

Fig. 2.1 Normally centred frontal chest radiograph. The medial borders of the clavicles (mbc) are equidistant from the spinous processes (sp).

7

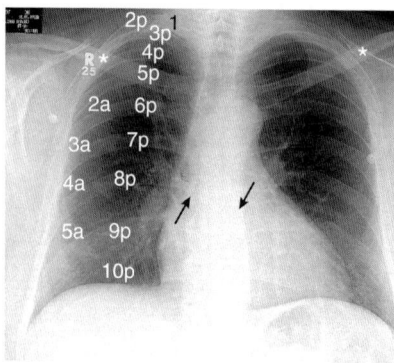

Fig. 2.2 Normal inspiration and penetration on the frontal chest radiograph. There are 10 ribs visible posteriorly (p) and 5 ribs anteriorly (a) in the mid-clavicular line (*). The vertebral column is discernible behind the heart (arrows).

Inspiration

On a standard frontal chest radiograph, inspiratory effort is measured at the level of the mid-clavicular line. Standard measurements would be 10 ribs visible posteriorly, and 5–7 ribs anteriorly (**Fig. 2.2**).

Penetration

With adequate penetration the thoracic vertebrae should be projected through the heart border and the intervertebral discs should be barely discernible (**Fig. 2.2**).

THE HEART AND CARDIAC SILHOUETTE

Heart size

The transverse diameter of the heart should be less than half the maximum chest diameter. This is confirmed using the cardiothoracic ratio (CTR). This ratio is defined as the distance between the apex and the extreme right edge of the heart border, divided by the maximum transverse diameter of the chest (**Fig. 2.3**).

The heart borders

On the frontal radiograph, the heart borders are as follows (**Fig. 2.4**):

Left heart border

Superior: Aortic knuckle
Pulmonary trunk
Inferior: Left ventricle

Right heart border

Superior: Superior vena cava
Right atrium
Inferior vena cava

The heart valves
Identification of the valves

On the anterior projection, the aortic valve overlies the spine, lying at the junction of the lower and middle thirds of the cardiac silhouette. The mitral valve lies to the left of the midline, usually below a line between the right anterior cardiophrenic angle and the left hilum (**Fig. 2.5a**).

On the lateral projection, the aortic valve lies above a line between the carina and the anterior cardiophrenic angle. The mitral valve lies below it and the tricuspid valve is bisected by it (**Fig. 2.5b**).

The diameter of the cardiac valves is inversely proportional to the pressure across them. Therefore the aortic valve is the smallest, then pulmonary, mitral and tricuspid (see **Fig. 2.6**).

Cardiomegaly

Cardiomegaly is present when the CTR exceeds 0.55. Selective chamber enlargement can occur.

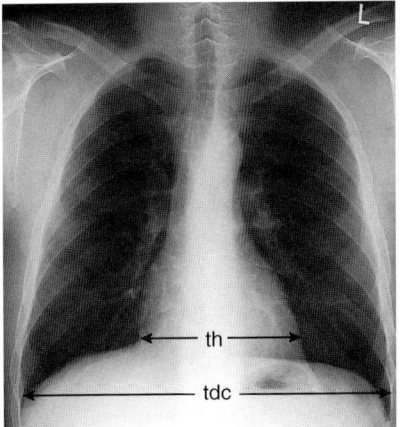

Fig. 2.3 Normal cardiothoracic ratio. The maximum transverse diameter of the heart (th) should be less than half of the transverse diameter of the chest (tdc).

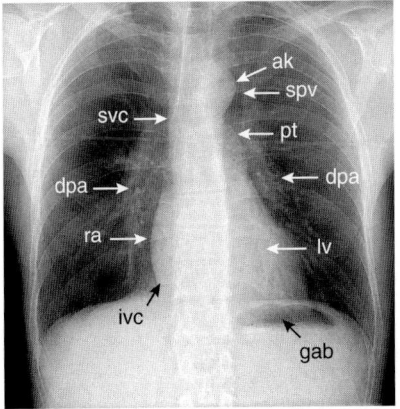

Fig. 2.4 The normal cardiac silhouette. spv: superior pulmonary vein, dpa: descending pulmonary artery, ra: right atrium, lv: left ventricle, pt: pulmonary trunk, ak: aortic knuckle, gab: gastric air bubble, svc: superior vena cava, ivc: inferior vena cava.

Left atrial enlargement

On the anterior projection, several signs have been described (**Fig. 2.7**).

1. There is a double density produced by the left atrial contour within the right atrial shadow. (Note that the left atrium does not extend inferiorly to the diaphragm)

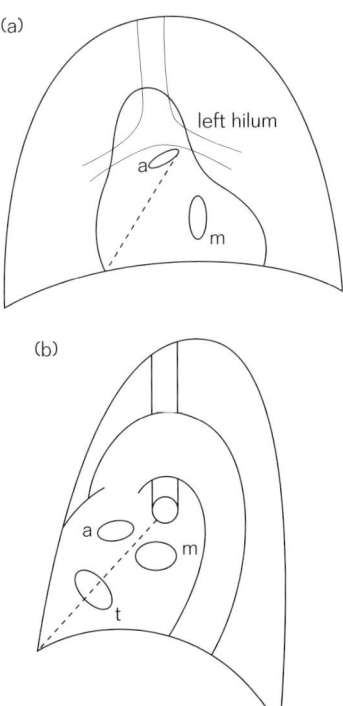

Fig. 2.5 Diagram demonstrating the position of the heart valves on (**a**) the frontal and (**b**) the lateral chest radiograph. a: aortic valve, m: mitral valve, t: tricuspid valve.

2. A line between the mid-border of the left atrium and the left bronchus is less than or equal to 7 cm
3. The sub-carinal angle is greater than 90°
4. There is enlargement of the left atrial appendage.

Left ventricular enlargement

On the anterior view, the enlarged left ventricle displaces the apex downwards and to the left (**Fig. 2.8**).

Right atrial enlargement

The right heart border becomes convex and moves to the right.

Right ventricular enlargement

Unless the right ventricle is very large, it does not normally form part of the heart

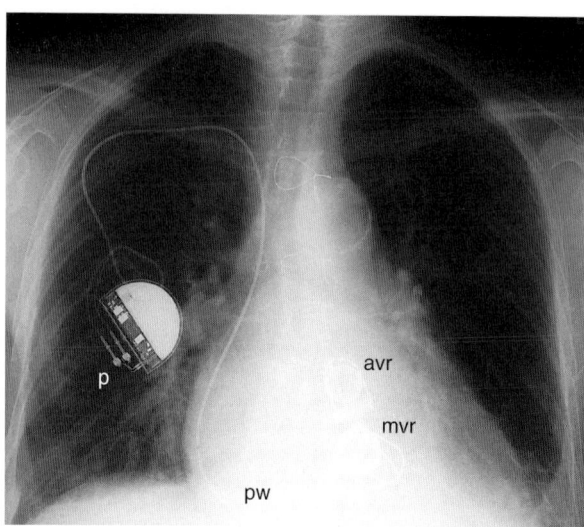

Fig. 2.6 Prosthetic mitral and aortic heart valves: frontal chest radiograph.
p: Pacemaker, pw: pacing wire, avr: aortic valve replacement, mvp: mitral valve replacement.

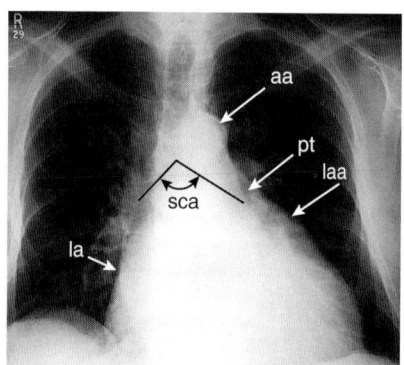

Fig. 2.7 Radiographic appearances of left atrial enlargement. Note splaying of the subcarinal angle (sca), the double atrial shadow caused by the enlarged left atrium (la), and the prominent left atrial appendage (laa). aa: aortic arch, pt: pulmonary trunk, sca: subcarinal angle.

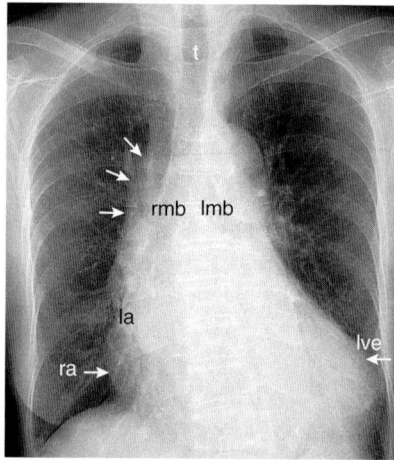

Fig. 2.8 Radiographic appearances of left ventricular enlargement. The underlying pathology was aortic valve stenosis, and post-stenotic dilatation (arrows) is present (confirmed at surgery). Left atrial enlargement is also present. t: trachea, lmb: left main bronchus, rmb: right main bronchus, ra: right atrium, la: left atrium, lve: left ventricular enlargement.

border. With right ventricular enlargement, the left ventricle is pushed laterally, upturning the cardiac apex (**Fig. 2.9**).

On the lateral radiograph, the anterior border of the right ventricle often lies in close contact with the posterior border of the sternum. If the heart border makes contact with more than one-third of the sternum, this indicates right ventricular enlargement.

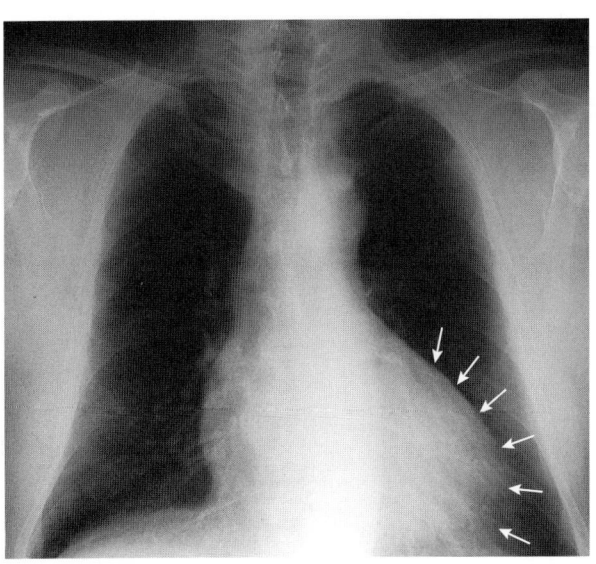

Fig. 2.9 Upturned cardiac apex in right ventricular enlargement (arrows).

PULMONARY VASCULARITY

Evaluation of the pulmonary vessels is essential in confirming cardiac failure and fluid overload

Normal vascularity

- No discrete vessels visible in the outer third of the lung

- Vascular predominance in the lower zones
- Vessels and bronchi are of equivalent cross-sectional diameter
- No Kerley B lines (basal subpleural interlobular lymphatic channels).

CARDIAC FAILURE

Cardiac failure is typically manifest by cardiomegaly (vide supra), increased pulmonary vascularity and air space changes in the lungs (vide infra).

Pulmonary venous hypertension

The earliest abnormality identified on an erect chest radiograph is vascular change, i.e. diversion of the blood flow to the upper lobes. This occurs at a pulmonary capillary wedge pressure (PCWP) of 12–19 mmHg and is manifest as an increase in vessel diameter of greater than 3 mm in the first intercostal interspace. There should also be a concomitant decrease in the size of the lower lobe vessels (**Fig. 2.10**).

As the PCWP rises above 19 mmHg, interstitial changes develop. The bronchial wall, normally pencil-thin in cross-section, becomes 'fuzzy', with indistinct margins. This is called *peribronchial cuffing*. Other

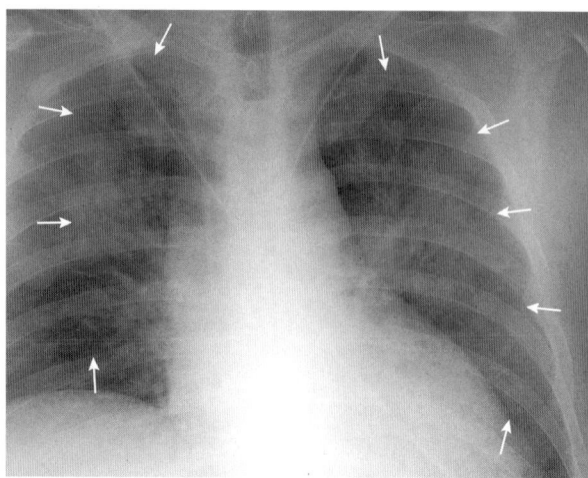

Fig. 2.10 Appearances in early cardiac failure. There are bilateral interstitial perihilar shadows present (arrows). These features are typical of early cardiac failure.

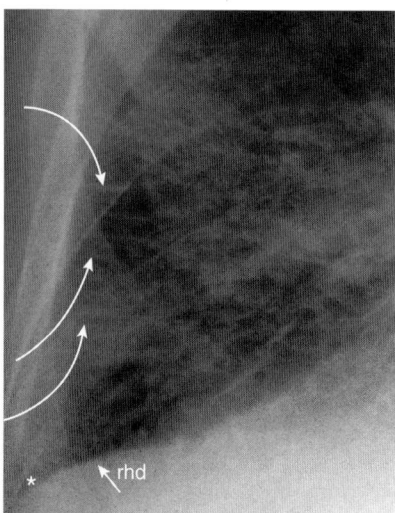

Fig. 2.11 Kerley B lines (curved arrows). rhd: right hemi-diaphragm, *: right costophrenic angle.

radiological signs include thickening of the lung fissures and Kerley B lines (1–2 cm horizontal peripheral linear densities seen at the lower lateral lung margins), which represent interlobular septal oedema (**Fig. 2.11**).

At PCWPs above 25 mmHg, air space changes (i.e. bronchograms – see p13) develop. These are typically perihilar and are described as *the bat's wings* (**Fig. 2.12**).

Radiographic features in chronic congestive heart failure occur at pressures 5 mmHg higher than with acute congestive heart failure.

PARENCHYMAL LUNG DISEASE

Aside from focal masses, two main patterns of pathology affect the lung parenchyma. These are diseases of the interstices and diseases of the airways.

Interstitial lung disease

The interstices, which surround the acini, are essentially septa, containing veins and lymphatic channels. Diseases affecting the interstices may do so by blocking these channels, e.g. cardiac failure (veins) and lymphangitis carcinomatosa (lymphatics), or by inducing a form of inflammatory response within them, e.g. asbestosis. As the interstices are lines and interlocking junctions, such diseases are manifested by

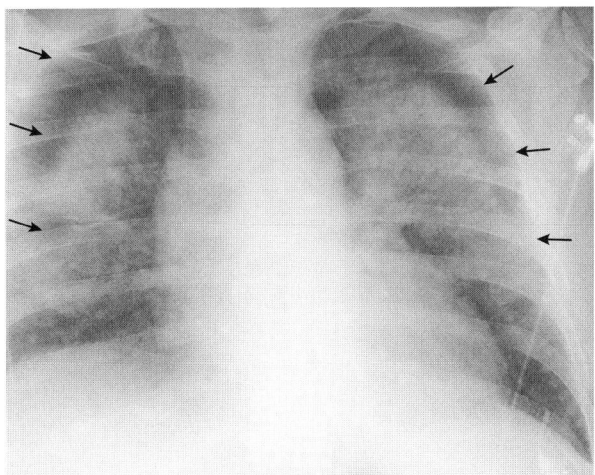

Fig. 2.12 Cardiac failure: pulmonary oedema (arrows). The earlier perihilar interstitial markings have now evolved into discrete 'bat's wing' shadows typical of pulmonary oedema.

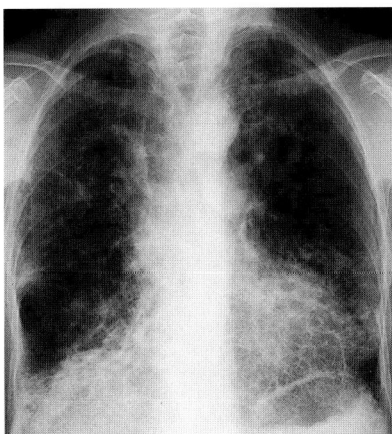

Fig. 2.13 Reticulonodular pattern in interstitial lung disease. Look for lines and dots. (The underlying cause was rheumatoid lung.)

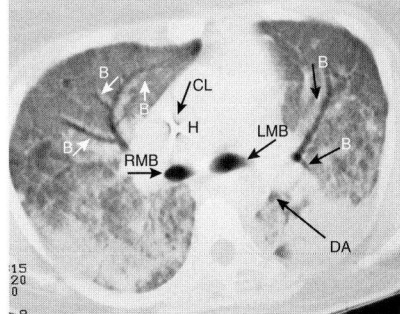

Fig. 2.14 The air bronchogram in consolidation. Look for bronchograms. (The underlying cause was ARDS. B: bronchus, H: heart, RMB: right main bronchus, LMB: left main bronchus, CL: central line, DA: descending aorta.

exaggeration of these features, producing the so-called *reticulonodular* or 'honeycombing' pattern of disease, recognizable by lines and dots (**Fig. 2.13**).

Airway disease

Airway disease produces *bronchograms*, i.e. the branching pattern of the air-filled bronchus seen against a background of greyer, consolidated acini. The archetypal

example is consolidation, e.g. produced by pneumonia (**Fig. 2.14**).

Pneumonia

Pneumonia is a form of air space consolidation, and therefore presents radiologically as a bronchogram. Clearly, as the disease progresses the bronchi occlude and there is segmental or lobar collapse.

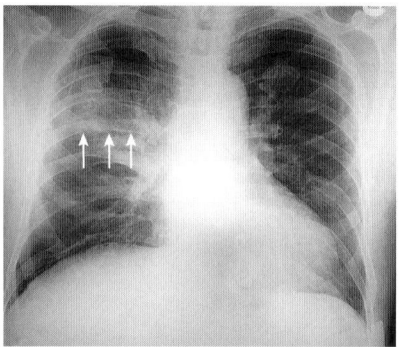

Fig. 2.15 Right upper lobe consolidation. There is an area of increased density in the right chest. The lower border of this area is the minor fissure. This confirms the anatomical location of the consolidation as the right upper lobe.

Identification of the affected lobe

Identifying the affected lobe depends on loss of the appropriate silhouette on the chest radiograph. The heart, mediastinum and the hemidiaphragms are identifiable on the chest film because they are surrounded by air in the acini. Should this air interface be lost, then that silhouette is lost or effaced (see **Table 2.1** and **Figs 2.15–2.21**).

Radiographic patterns in specific pneumonias

The appearances in pneumonia can be non-specific, but there are some clues, as shown in **Table 2.2** (p. 17).

Table 2.1 Identification of lobar consolidation/collapse on the frontal chest radiograph	
Consolidated/collapsed area	**Silhouette lost is:**
Right upper lobe	Right upper mediastinum[a]
Right middle lobe	Right heart border
Right lower lobe	Right hemidiaphragm
Left upper lobe	Aortic knuckle
Lingula	Left heart border
Left lower lobe	Left hemidiaphragm

[a] The right upper lobe, when consolidated, has a horizontal lower margin produced by the minor fissure.

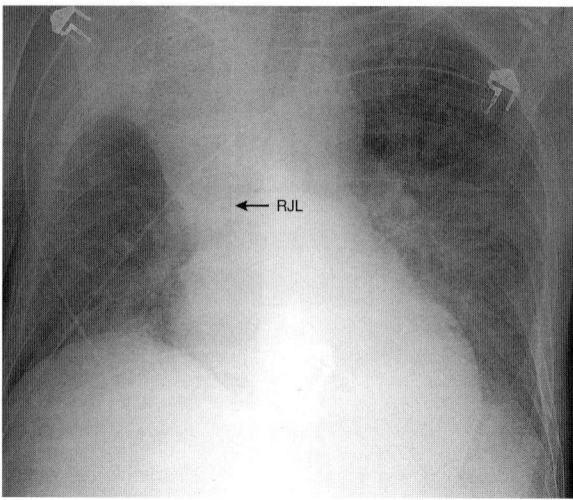

← RJL

Fig. 2.16(a) Right upper lobe collapse: pre-therapy. The collapsed right upper lobe is identified as an area of increased density in the right upper chest. Note there is no mass effect, i.e. no contralateral displacement of the mediastinum to the left, as might be the case with an intrathoracic/pleural bleed. RJL: right jugular line.

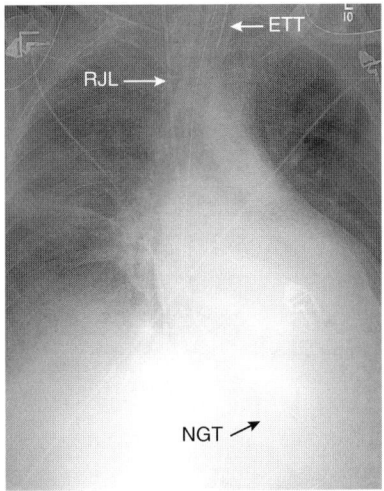

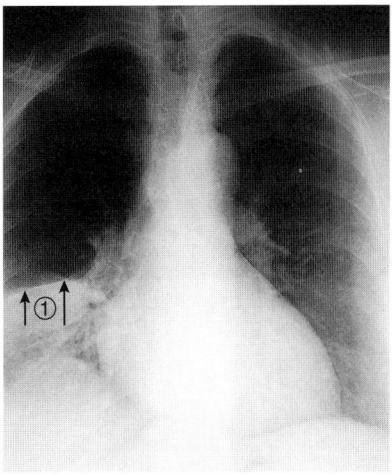

Fig. 2.16(b) Right upper lobe collapse: post-therapy. 12 hours after physiotherapy the lobe has re-expanded. RJL: right jugular line, ETT: endotracheal tube, NGT: nasogastric tube.

Fig. 2.17 Right middle lobe consolidation. Note that the consolidated lung is bounded superiorly by the minor fissure (①), thus confirming the anatomical location of the consolidation as being in the right middle lobe.

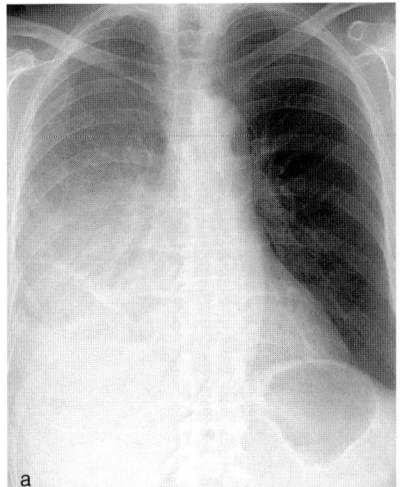

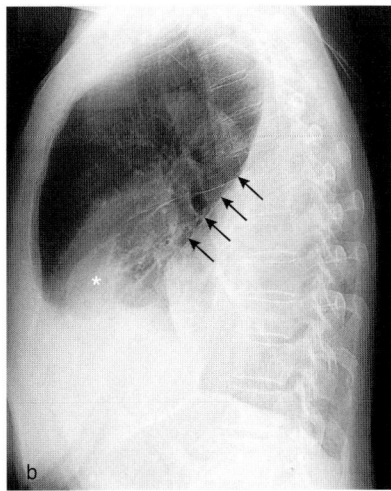

Fig. 2.18(a) Right lower lobe consolidation, anterior chest radiograph. There is increased density in the right lung with loss of the right hemidiaphragm. **(b)** The diagnosis is confirmed on this lateral radiograph by the consolidation posterior to the major fissure (arrows). Note there is also subtle right middle lobe consolidation (*).

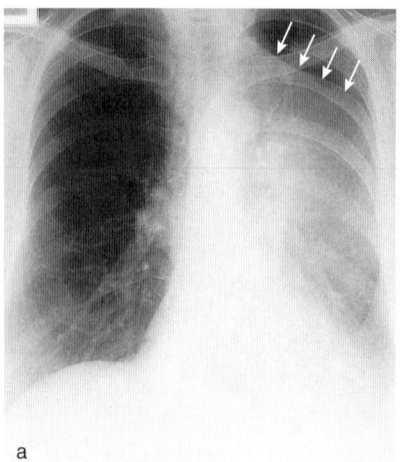 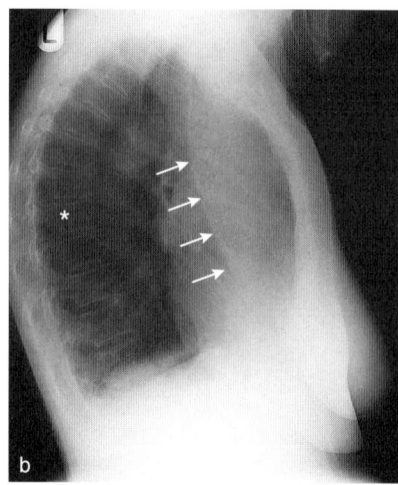

Fig. 2.19 Left upper lobe collapse: (**a**) Frontal chest radiograph. The upper margin of the collapsed left upper lobe (arrows) obscures the aortic arch. (**b**) Lateral chest radiograph. The collapsed left upper lobe 'falls forward' (arrows). Note the compensatory overinflation of the left lower lobe (*).

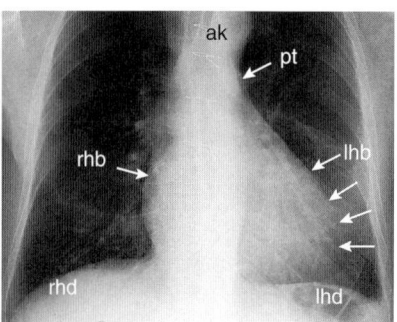 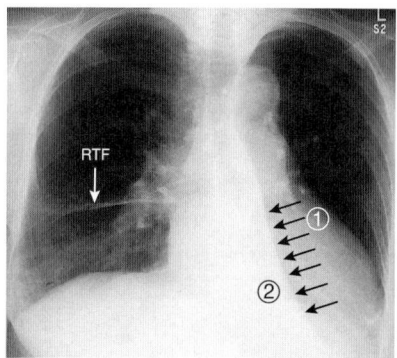

Fig. 2.20 Lingular consolidation, the silhouette of the cardia apex is missing. ak: aortic knuckle, pt: pulmonary trunk, rhb: right heart border, lhb: left heart border, lhd: left hemidiaphragm, rhd: right hemidiaphragm.

Fig. 2.21 Left lower lobe collapse. Note the double density behind the heart (①) and the effacement of the medial portion of the left hemidiaphragm (②). Note also the prominence of the right transverse fissure (RTF): this suggests previous atelectasis or inflammatory change.

PULMONARY EMBOLISM

The plain chest radiograph is unreliable in diagnosing pulmonary embolism. A normal radiograph does not exclude the diagnosis. The main role of the chest radiograph is to exclude other pathology.

Plain radiographs and pulmonary embolism

There are three eponymous signs described on the plain chest radiograph: the Westermark sign, Chang's sign and Hampton's hump.

Table 2.2 Radiographic patterns in specific pneumonias	
Radiographic sign	**Pneumonia due to:**
Round pneumonia	Pneumococcus (The commonest community-acquired pneumonia)
Lobar enlargement	Staphylococcus Klebsiella Tuberculosis Haemophilus
Cavitation	Staphylococcus *Streptococcus pyogenes* Klebsiella Tuberculosis Gram-negative organisms
Hilar lymphadenopathy	Tuberculosis Fungi Mycoplasma Viral

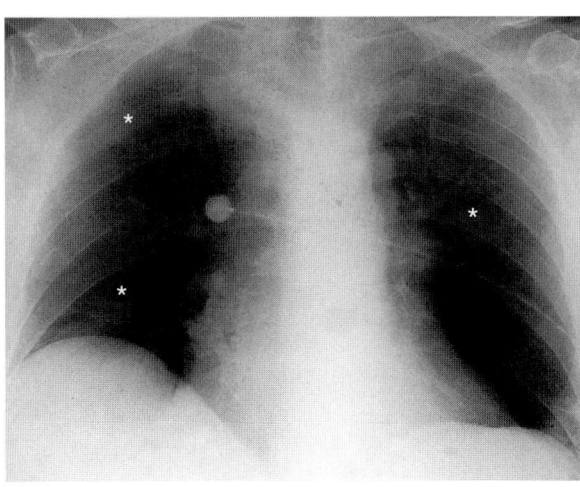

Fig. 2.22 Pulmonary embolism: the Westermark sign. There is markedly reduced pulmonary vascularity in almost all of the right lung and most of the left lung.

The Westermark sign

This is the finding of oligaemia (or relatively increased darkness) on the affected side (**Fig. 2.22**).

Chang's sign

This is evidence of pulmonary artery enlargement proximal to the embolism (**Fig. 2.23**).

17

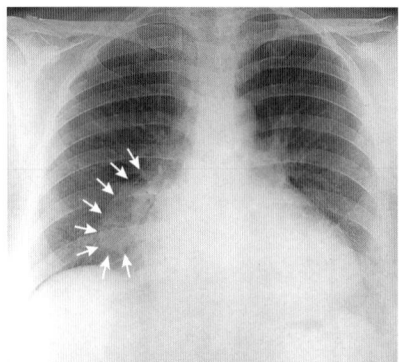

Fig. 2.23 Pulmonary embolism: Chang's sign. The right descending pulmonary artery is enlarged secondary to the embolus lodged distally.

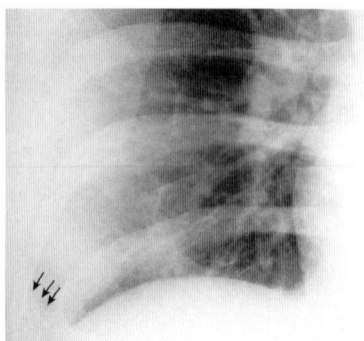

Fig. 2.24 Pulmonary embolism: Hampton's hump.

Hampton's hump

This is a triangular area of consolidation, usually found at the right lung base, near the costophrenic angle, representing pulmonary infarction (**Fig. 2.24**).

Pulmonary embolism and computed tomography

Computed tomographic angiography, a technique using helical CT scanning, has recently been developed as a non-invasive alternative to conventional pulmonary angiography. The emboli are seen as dark filling defects within the bright blood-filled vessels (**Fig. 2.25**).

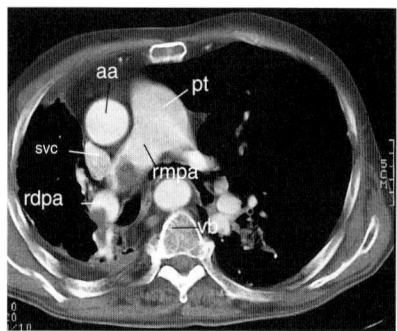

Fig. 2.25 Pulmonary embolism: CT demonstrating embolus in the right main and descending pulmonary artery. The embolic material is seen as filling defects in the right main pulmonary artery (rmpa) and the right descending pulmonary artery (rdpa). aa: ascending aorta, svc: superior vena cava, pt: pulmonary trunk, vb: vertebral body.

CHEST TRAUMA

Tubes and lines

Endotracheal tube

The tip of the endotracheal tube should lie 2–5 cm above the level of the carina. A tube placed at the carina may, with respiration, slide into one of the main bronchi, usually the right, thus occluding the other (**Figs 2.26 and 2.27**).

Nasogastric tube

The tip of the nasogastric (NG) tube should lie in the stomach. On the chest radiograph, the tip of the NG tube should be seen lying in the left upper quadrant of the abdomen (**Figs 2.28 and 2.29**).

Central venous lines

Central venous (CVP) lines are usually inserted via the jugular or subclavian

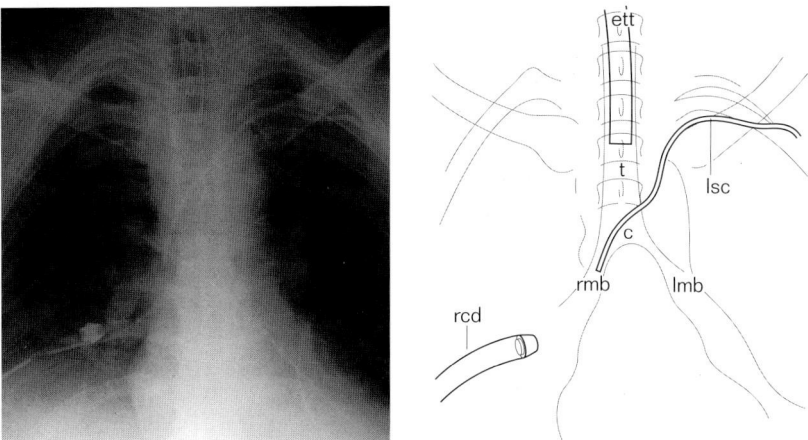

Fig. 2.26 Correct position of endotracheal tube (ett). t: trachea, c: carina, rmb: right main bronchus, lmb: left main bronchus, rcd: right chest drain, lsc: left subclavia catheter.

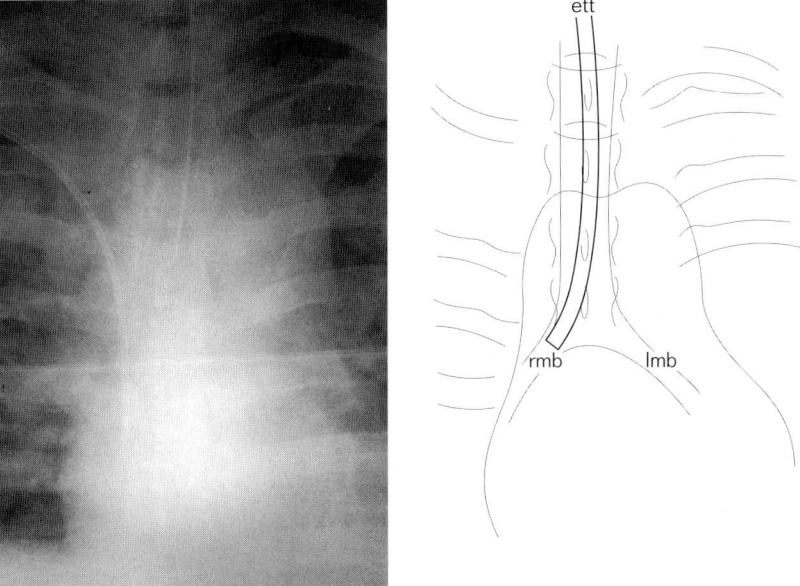

Fig. 2.27 Endotracheal tube tip lying in right main bronchus (rmb). lmb: left main bronchus.

route. The tip of the central line should lie at the junction of the right atrium and the superior vena cava. On the chest radiograph, the tip of the CVP line should lie inferomedial to the anterior portion of the right first rib (**Fig. 2.26**).

Pulmonary arterial catheter

Swan–Ganz (central arterial) catheters are usually inserted via the jugular vein and the tip of the catheter should lie wedged in the pulmonary artery. The tip of the catheter in the central right or left

19

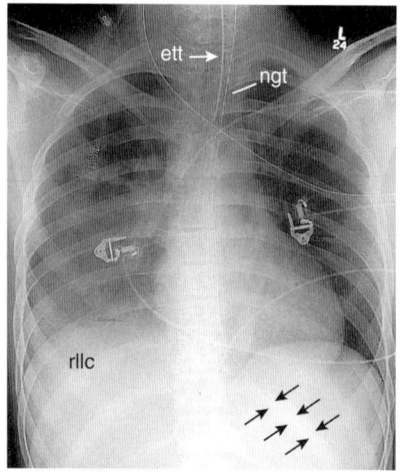

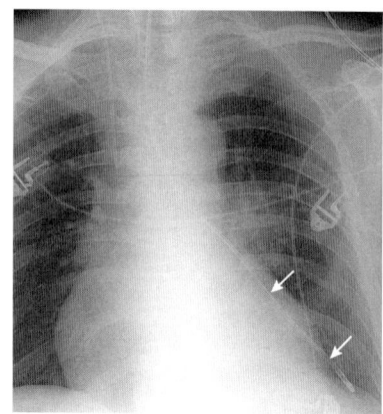

Fig. 2.29 Nasogastric tube (arrowed) misplaced in the left lower lobe bronchus.

Fig. 2.28 Nasogastric tube (ngt) in correct position (arrows). Note that there is right lower lobe consolidation with loss of the lateral position of the right hemidiaphragm. ett: endotracheal tube, rllc: right lower lobe consolidation.

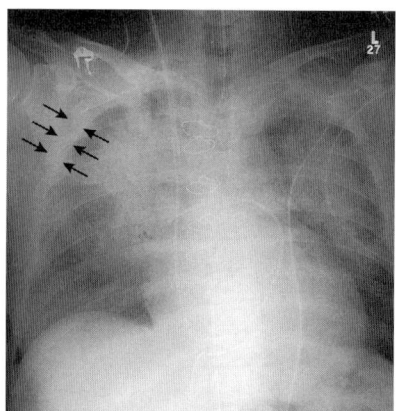

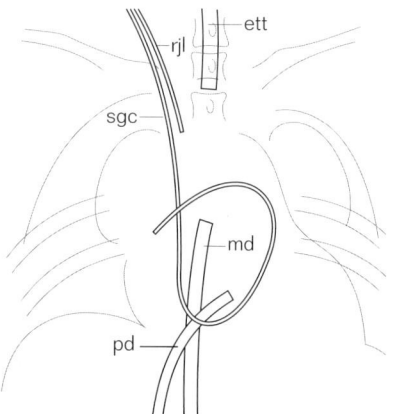

Fig. 2.30 Swan-Ganz pulmonary artery catheter (sgc). This radiograph also illustrates the typical drains and tubes used post-cardiac surgery. Note the 'bat's wing' appearance of the perihilar shadows, indicating cardiac failure. In addition there is a subtle right-sided pleural fluid collection (arrows). ett: endotracheal tube, rjl: right jugular central venous line, md: mediastinal drain, pd: pericardial drain.

pulmonary artery should be less than 2 cm lateral to the hilum (**Fig. 2.30**).

Intra-aortic balloon pump catheter

The tip of the aortic balloon pump catheter should lie below the left subclavian artery and above the renal arteries. It may be identified by its radiopaque tip (**Fig. 2.31**), and also by the carbon dioxide gas which inflates the balloon during diastole.

Note: Following line placement, it is routine practice to check position and

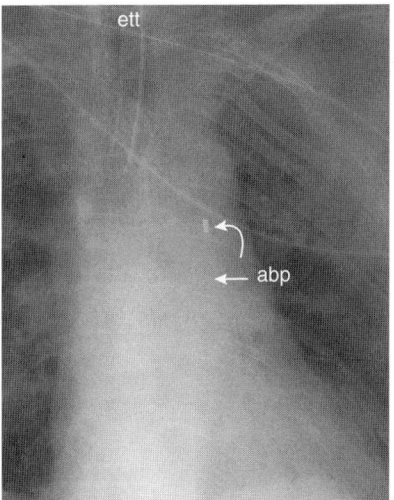

Fig. 2.31 Radiograph appearances of intra-aortic balloon pump catheter (abp). The tip of the pump (curved arrow) should lie below the left subclavian artery. Note also the correctly positioned endotracheal tube (ett).

exclude pneumothorax with an erect chest radiograph.

Pneumothorax

A pneumothorax can be identified on both the routine anterior and the supine chest radiographs.

On the erect radiograph this is more clearly identified on the expiratory film, when the relatively increased pressure within the pleural space maximizes the size of the pneumothorax (**Fig. 2.32a, b; p. 22**). It is crucial to recognize radiographic signs of tension:

1. Flattening of the hemidiaphragm, especially in ventilated patients
2. Mediastinal shift to the opposite side.

On the supine film, free pleural air will lie anterior to the lung and therefore the pattern is different. The following are signs of pneumothorax on a supine film

(**Fig. 2.33a, b; p. 22**):

1. Deep costophrenic sulcus
2. Sharp cardiac outline
3. .Cardiac fat pad clearly seen
4. Transradiant hypochondrium.

Pleural blood and effusions

The radiographic appearances depend on whether the film has been obtained in the routine anterior erect, or supine position.

Erect film

The pleural fluid tracks to the lung base, often obscuring the hemidiaphragm, and producing a meniscus at the chest wall interface (**Fig. 2.34; p. 23**).

Supine film

Here, the pleural fluid tracks posteriorly along the posterior pleural space towards the apex. This has a 'veiled' appearance on the radiograph, making the affected side 'greyer' than the normal side (**Figs 2.35 and 2.36; p. 23**). Dramatic improvement is achieved with the insertion of a chest drain.

The acutely injured lung

These injuries are usually the result of crush or rapid deceleration injuries to the chest. It is important to recognize that the initial, or 'index', chest radiograph may be normal.

Pulmonary contusion

These occur rapidly after injury, may be associated with myocardial contusions, and can be remembered by the 72-hour rule: *Contusions appear within 72 hours and disappear after a further 72 hours.*

Pulmonary contusions (**Fig. 2.37**):

- Occur within hours of trauma
- Distribution in lung reflects the area of injury
- Tend to be poorly defined
- Cross fissures
- Typically resolve within 72 hours.

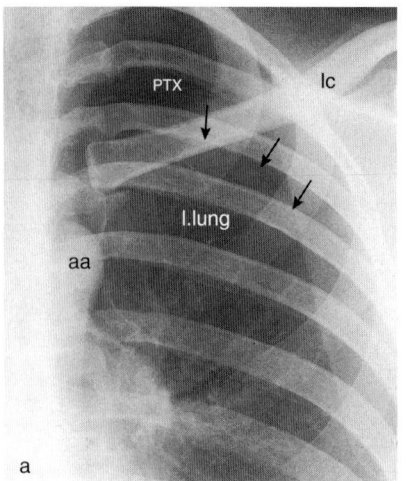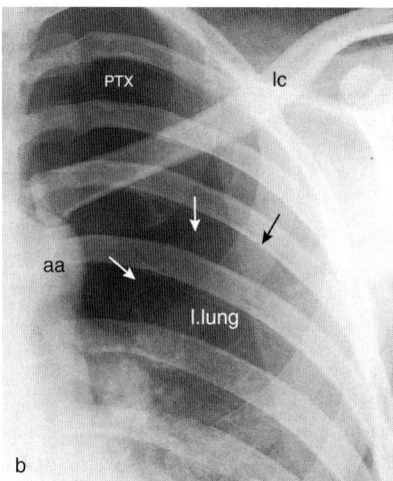

Fig. 2.32 Pneumothorax (PTX) on (**a**) inspiratory and (**b**) expiratory radiographs. Note that the pneumothorax is much more clearly appreciated on the expiratory view. aa: aortic arch, l. lung: left lung, lc: left clavicle.

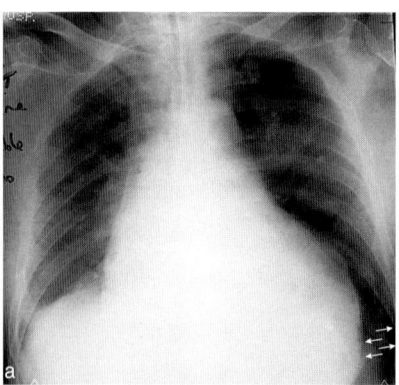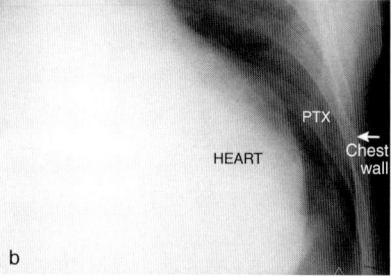

Fig. 2.33 Appearances of a pneumothorax on (**a**) the supine radiograph and (**b**) detail of the left costophrenic angle. PTX: pneumothorax.

Pneumatocele

Pneumatoceles:

- Occur several hours after the injury
- Are caused by shock waves tearing the lung parenchyma
- The lung retracts back from the torn surface
- Air escapes into the new space
- Resolution is within weeks–months of the injury.

Pulmonary haematoma

Pulmonary haematoma (**Fig. 2.38a, b**):

- Usually appear after 3 days
- Are round with discrete margins
- May take up to 6 months to disappear!

Aortic injury

Injury to the thoracic aorta is an important complication of blunt thoracic trauma

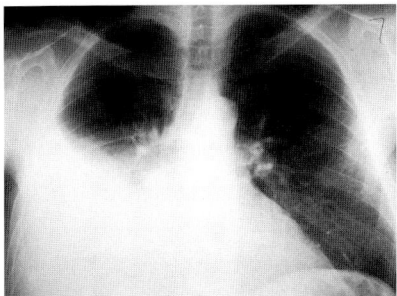

Fig. 2.34 Large right-sided pleural effusion (erect chest radiograph). The lack of contra-lateral mediastinal shift indicates underlying right segmental/lobar lung collapse.

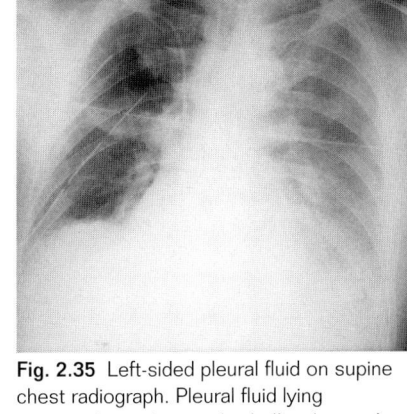

Fig. 2.35 Left-sided pleural fluid on supine chest radiograph. Pleural fluid lying posteriorly produces a 'veiled' or 'ground glass' appearance to the left lung.

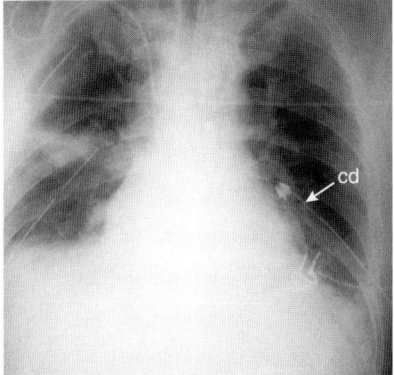

Fig. 2.36 The same patient as Fig. 2.35 following left chest drain placement (cd). Both lungs are equally transradiant.

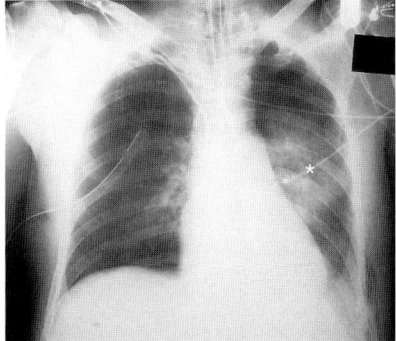

Fig. 2.37 Radiographic appearance of a pulmonary contusion in the left lung (*). Note the associated loss of the left hemidiaphragm silhouette.

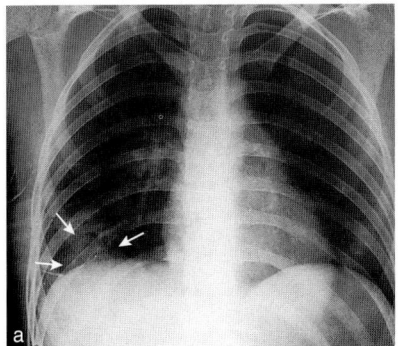

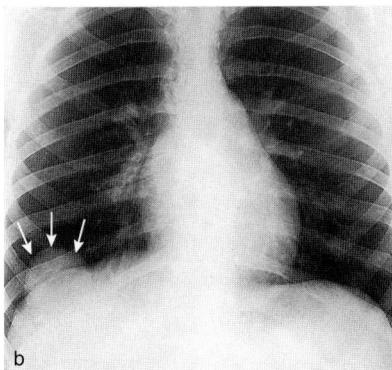

Fig. 2.38 Pulmonary haematoma (**a**) following road traffic accident. Patchy obfuscation can be seen at the right base (arrows). The area at the right base evolved into a rounded lesion. (**b**) 28 days afterwards, the haematoma can be seen (arrows). This mass resolved progressively over several weeks.

with a high morbidity and mortality. The site of injury is typically at the level of the aortic isthmus, i.e. just distal to the left subclavian artery where the 'free' aortic arch joins the restrained thoracic aorta. Shear forces are maximal at this point. Radiographic evidence of aortic injury is considered in the list below with examples (**Figs 2.39–2.41**).

Radiographic signs of aortic injury

Features due to the haematoma formation

- Mediastinal diameter greater than 8 cm
- Obscured descending aortic contour
- Mediastinum : thoracic ratio greater than 0.25

Features due to the mass effect of the haematoma on adjacent structures

- Inferior displacement of the left main bronchus (⩾ 40° from the horizontal)
- Trachea and nasogastric tube displaced to the right

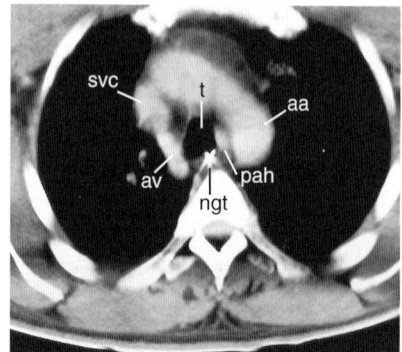

Fig. 2.40 Aortic dissection: para-aortic mediastinal blood on CT. svc: superior vena cava, t: trachea, aa: aortic arch, pah: periaortic haematoma/blood, ngt: nasogastric tube, av: azygos vein.

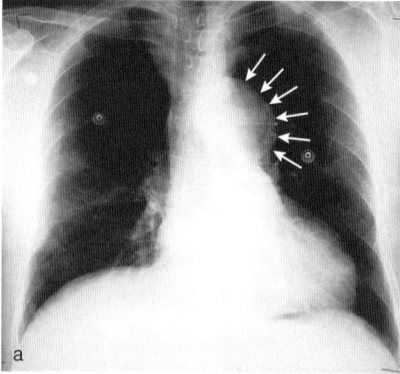

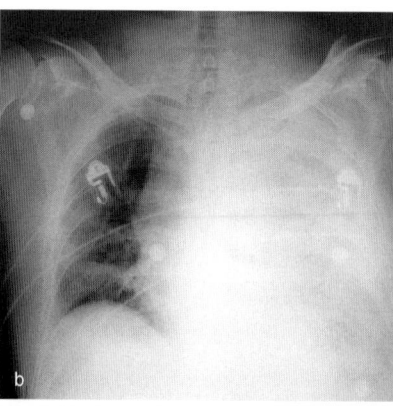

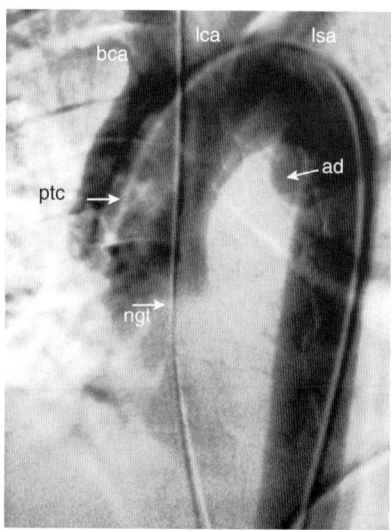

Fig. 2.41 Aortic dissection: angiographic confirmation. (Same patient as Fig. 2.40.) bca: brachiocephalic artery, lca: left carotid artery, lsa: left subclavian artery, ptc: pigtail catheter, ad: aortic dissection, ngt: nasogastric tube.

Fig. 2.39 Aortic dissection: (**a**) widened mediastinum on chest radiograph (arrows) and (**b**) post-rupture. Blood fills the left chest.

Features due to leakage of blood elsewhere

- Apical capping
- Haemorrhage into the pleural space causing:

1. loss of the hemidiaphragm and costophrenic angle on erect film
2. a ground glass appearance to the affected side ('veiling') on the supine film.

ADULT RESPIRATORY DISTRESS SYNDROME

Adult respiratory distress syndrome (ARDS) is a protean response to many types of lung insult. The diagnosis is made by satisfying four criteria:

- Appropriate history
- Consistent X-ray appearances (see below)
- Ratio of $PaO_2:FiO_2$ less than 200
- Pulmonary arterial wedge pressure less than 18 mmHg.

In clinical practice, often there is considerable diagnostic dilemma distinguishing ARDS from cardiac failure (**Figs 2.42–2.44**). **Table 2.3** lists some of the main discriminating signs.

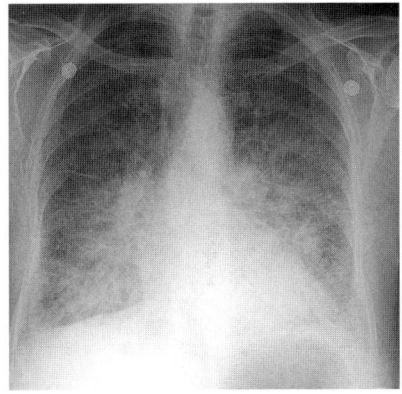

Fig. 2.42 Cardiac failure.

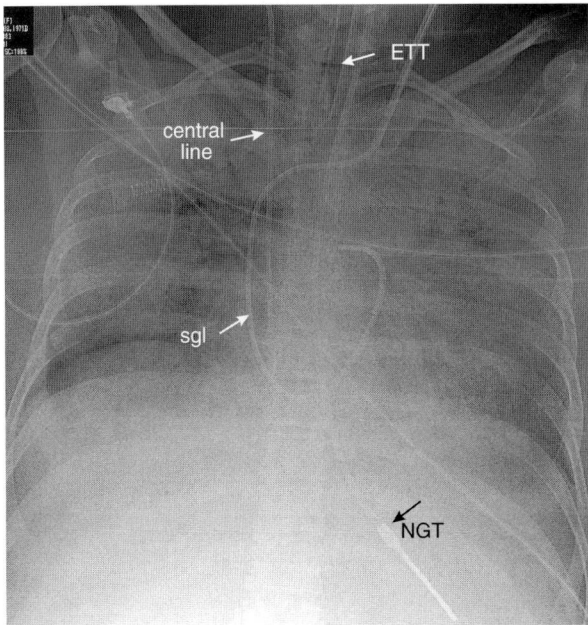

central line

ETT

sgl

NGT

Fig. 2.43 Adult respiratory distress syndrome. ETT: endotracheal tube, sgl: Swan-Ganz line, NGT: nasogastric tube.

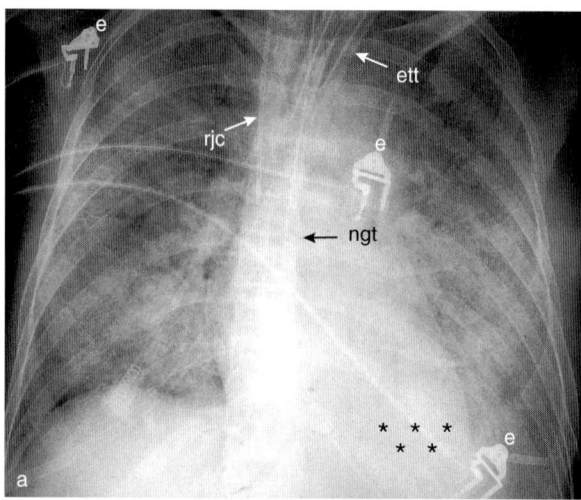

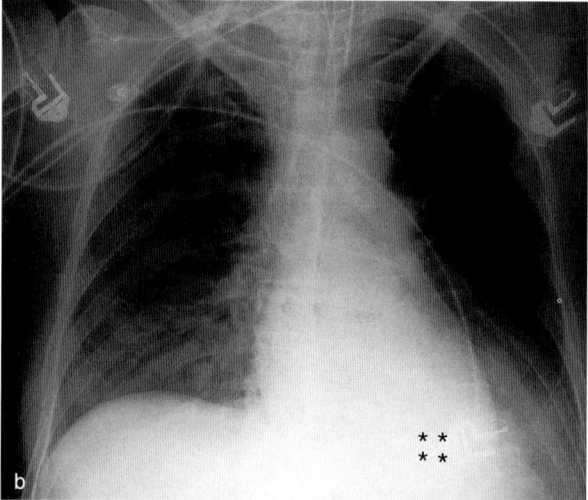

Fig. 2.44 Adult respiratory distress syndrome. (a) There is universal ground glass opacification of both lungs. There is also left lower lobe consolidation manifested by loss of the left hemidiaphragm silhouette (**). Compare these appearances with (b) the ICU chest radiograph taken 3 days earlier. There is left lower lobe collapse (**) but the remaining airways are clear. ett: endotracheal tube, rjc: right jugular catheter, ngt: nasogastric tube, e: ECG electrodes.

Table 2.3 Discriminating signs for ARDS and cardiac failure on the chest radiograph

Cardiac failure	ARDS
Rapid evolution	Slow evolution
X-ray appearances are concurrent with the clinical appearances	X-ray appearances lag behind the clinical appearances
Normal heart size	Cardiomegaly
Central distribution	Global distribution

Table 2.3 contd.	
Bronchograms rare	Bronchograms common
Pulmonary vascularity increased	Pulmonary vascularity normal
Upper zone diversion of blood	No upper zone diversion
Kerley B lines	No Kerley B lines
Pleural effusions	No pleural effusions

THE PULMONARY MASS

The key to localization of the pulmonary mass on the frontal chest radiograph is to evaluate its relationship to the heart and mediastinum. Masses that obscure part of the cardiac silhouette or displace the hilar vessels lie in the same plane, i.e. the middle mediastinum. When the cardiac and hilar silhouettes are seen through the mass, the mass must lie in front of, or behind them.

The next step is to examine the ribs in the same area. If there is destruction, erosion or splaying of the ribs, the mass is posterior.

Examine the relationship to the clavicle. If the mass is seen through or above the clavicle, again it must be posteriorly placed.

Nipple shadows

It is not uncommon to identify the nipple shadows on the frontal chest radiograph. Occasionally, there may be concern that the focal area seen is not in fact innocent. The radiologist will then recommend repeating the examination with nipple

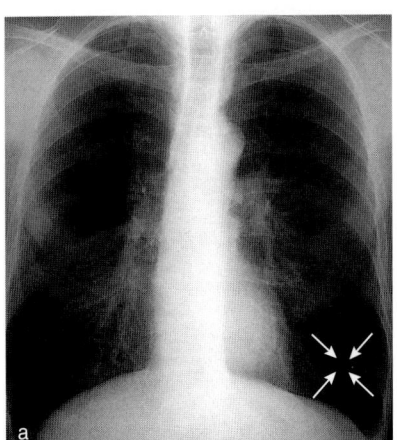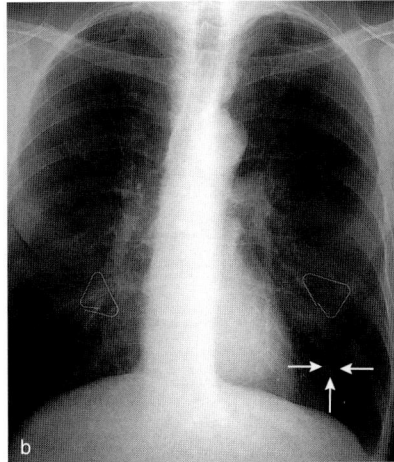

Fig. 2.45 Chest radiograph (**a**) demonstrating equivocal lesion at the left lung base and (**b**) following nipple marker placement. The lesion was intrapulmonary and proved to be a pulmonary metastasis.

markers in position. These are triangular metal strips (e.g. opened paperclip) taped around the nipple. Often it is helpful to repeat the examination in a different phase of respiration, as intrapulmonary masses will move whereas chest wall lesions will not (**Fig. 2.45a, b**).

Differential diagnosis of the mediastinal masses

It may be helpful to use mnemonics to remember these differential diagnoses. These are included now, in the parentheses.

Anterior mediastinal mass
(**Figs 2.46 and 2.47**)

(**The four 'Ts'**)

- **T**hymoma
- **T**eratoma
- **T**hyroid masses
- ('**T**errible'!) lymphoma

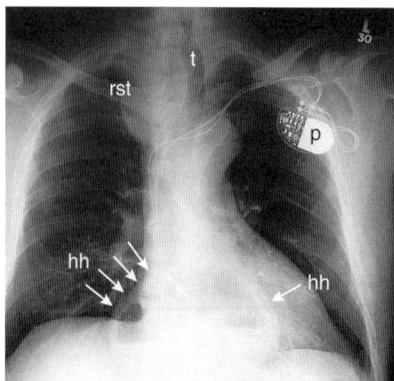

Fig. 2.46 Anterior mediastinal mass on chest radiograph. There is a mass lesion in the anterior and superior mediastinum. There is marked displacement of the trachea (t) to the left. The diagnosis was of retrosternal thyroid enlargement (rst). Note also the pacemaker (p) and a large fixed retrocardiac hiatus hernia (hh) with a fluid level.

Middle mediastinal mass
(**Figs 2.48 and 2.49**)

(**BLAB**)

- **B**ronchogenic carcinoma
- **L**ymphadenopathy
- **A**ortic aneurysm
- **B**ronchogenic cyst

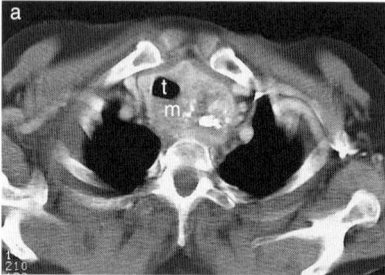

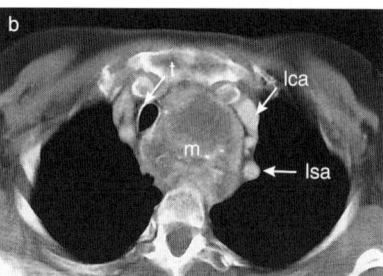

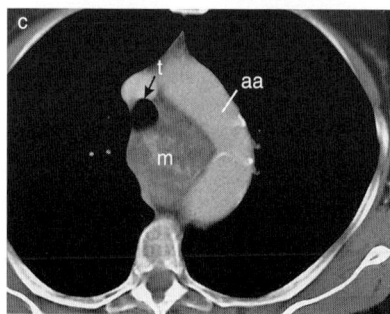

Fig. 2.47 Anterior mediastinal mass on CT. Retrosternal goitre with middle and posterior mediastinal extension. These three sections at the level of the suprasternal notch (**a**), great vessels (**b**) and aortic arch (**c**) demonstrate the inferior protrusion of the mass, with displacement and compression of the trachea (t). m: thyroid mass, lca: left carotid artery, lsa: left subclavian artery.

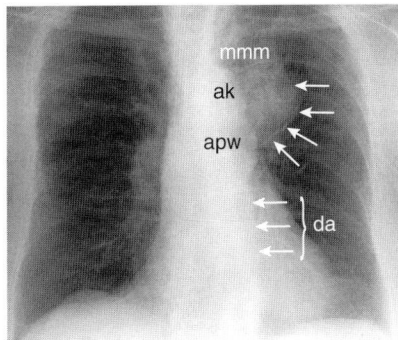

Fig. 2.48 Middle mediastinal mass (mmm) on chest radiograph. Although the aortic knuckle (ak) is still visible, there is a mass in the cardiopulmonary window (arrows) which obliterates a portion of the descending aorta. apw: aortopulmonary window, da: descending aorta.

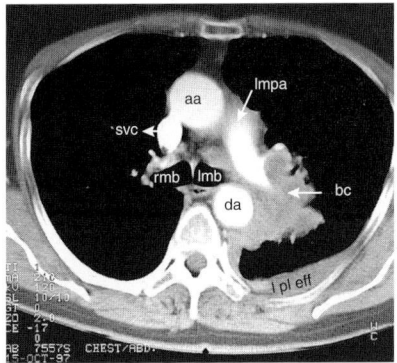

Fig. 2.49 Middle mediastinal mass on CT. The bronchogenic carcinoma (bc) envelops the left main pulmonary artery (lmpa) and abuts the descending aorta (da). svc: superior vena cava, aa: ascending aorta, rmb: right main bronchus, lmb: left main bronchus, l pl eff: left pleural effusion.

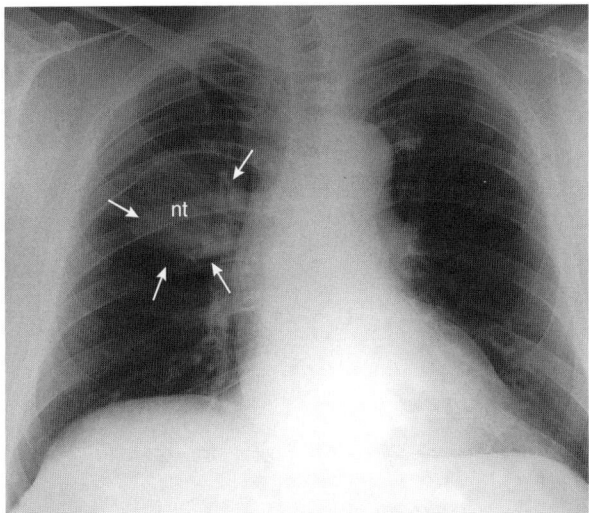

Fig. 2.50(a) Paraverebral mass on chest radiograph. Arrows indicate rib eroded by neurogenic tumour (nt).

Posterior mediastinal mass (DANE) and paravertebral (NOAH)

(DANE)

- **D**ilated oesophagus
- **A**ortic aneurysm/dissection
- **N**eurenteric cyst
- **E**nteric cyst

(NOAH) (Figs 2.50a and b)

- **N**eurogenic tumours
- **O**thers (ARE)
  - **a**nterior thoracic meningocele
  - **r**eticuloendothelial disorders
  - **e**xtramedullary haemopoiesis
- **A**bscess
- **H**ernia of Bochdalek

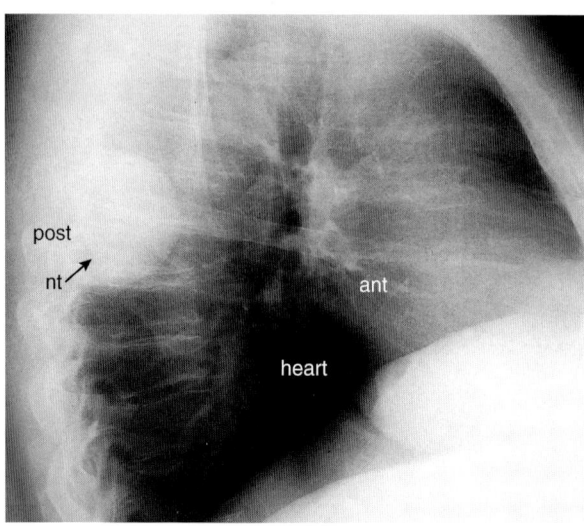

Fig. 2.50(b)
Paravertebral mass
on CT. nt: neurogenic
tumour.

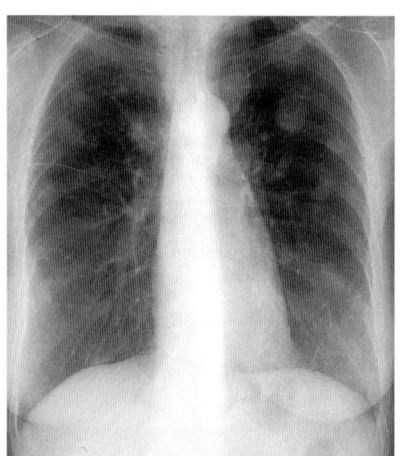

Fig. 2.51 Multiple pulmonary metastases.

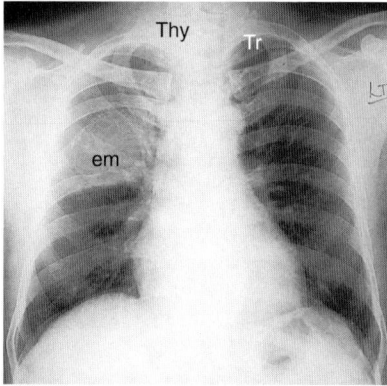

Fig. 2.52 Carcinoma of the thyroid with rib expansile metastasis (em). The right fifth rib is expanded and replaced by tumour. Note the tracheal displacement to the left (Tr) by a right lobar thyroid mass (Thy). (The diagnosis was of metastatic infiltration of the rib by a thyroid carcinoma.)

Pulmonary metastases

All malignant neoplasms have the potential to metastasize to lung, but over 80% arise from the breast, gastrointestinal or urogenital organs. The most common radiological pattern observed on the chest radiograph is that of multiple discrete nodules (**Fig. 2.51**). It is important to stress that this radiological pattern is non-specific, and the specificity of the diagnosis will depend on many factors, most notably, patient history.

Rib metastases

It is always prudent to scrutinize the ribs and bony skeleton for evidence of infiltration. **Figure 2.52** demonstrates an expansile lesion in the posterior aspect of a right-sided rib. The primary lesion was a carcinoma of the thyroid. Inspection of the suprasternal area demonstrates subtle tracheal displacement by the tumour.

Further Reading

Armstrong P, Wilson A G, Dee P, Hansell D M 1995 Imaging of diseases of the chest, 2nd edn. St Louis: Mosby.

Meholic A, Ketai L, Lofgren R 1996 Fundamentals of chest radiology. Philadelphia: WB Saunders.

Pare J A P, Fraser R G 1983 Synopsis of diseases of the chest, 2nd edn. Philadelphia: WB Saunders.

3 | Imaging in the Acute Abdomen

Topics included in this chapter

- Evaluation of the normal abdominal radiograph
- Intestinal obstruction
- Ileus and pseudo-obstruction
- Pneumoperitoneum
- Sepsis
- Miscellaneous acute abdominal pathological conditions

EVALUATION OF THE NORMAL ABDOMINAL RADIOGRAPH

The abdominal radiograph is one of the commonest films encountered in clinical practice. Consequently, a sound knowledge of the appearances of common pathological conditions is necessary.

Abdominal bowel gas patterns

Gas is normally present in the stomach and the colon (**Fig. 3.1**), but only a little is seen within the small bowel. More than two fluid levels in a *dilated* small bowel loop (i.e. calibre greater than 3.5 cm) are abnormal and may indicate paralytic ileus, pseudo-obstruction or obstruction. The valvulae conniventes are more obvious in the jejunum than in the ileum.

Although large bowel calibre is variable, a diameter of 6.5 cm is generally considered the upper limit of normal for the

transverse colon. Above this, underlying pathology should be considered. There is considerable variation in the caecal diameter but greater than 10 cm is abnormal and increases the risk of perforation.

The colonic haustra can sometimes form complete transverse bands but can usually be distinguished from the valvulae conniventes (**Fig. 3.2**) because they are thicker and further apart. Haustra may be absent from the descending colon and the sigmoid colon but can usually be

Small bowel dimensions		
	Jejunum	*Ileum*
Diameter	*3.5 cm*	*2.5 cm*
Wall thickness	*2.0 mm*	*2.0 mm*
Valvulae thickness	*2.5 mm*	*2.0 mm*

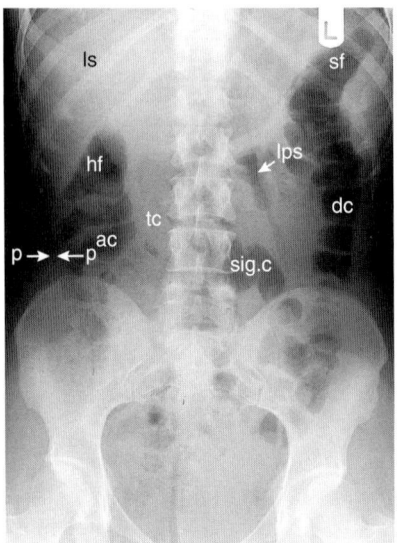

Fig. 3.1 Normal abdominal radiograph. ls: liver shadow, p→: properitoneal fat line, ac: ascending colon, hf: hepatic flexure, tc: transverse colon, sf: splenic flexure, dc: descending colon, sig.c: sigmoid colon, lps: left psoas shadow.

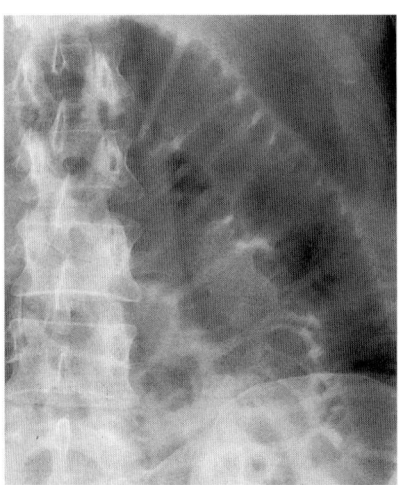

Fig. 3.2 Valvulae conniventes.

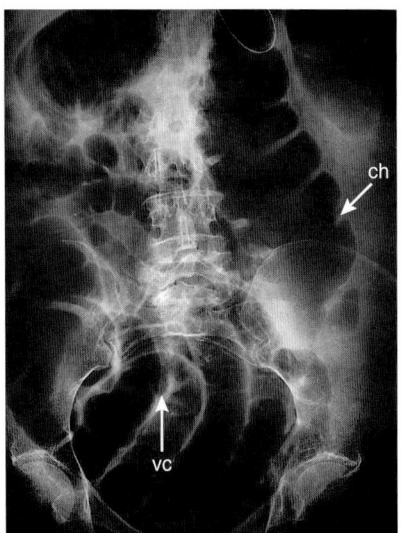

Fig. 3.3 Colonic haustra (ch) and valvulae conniventes (vc).

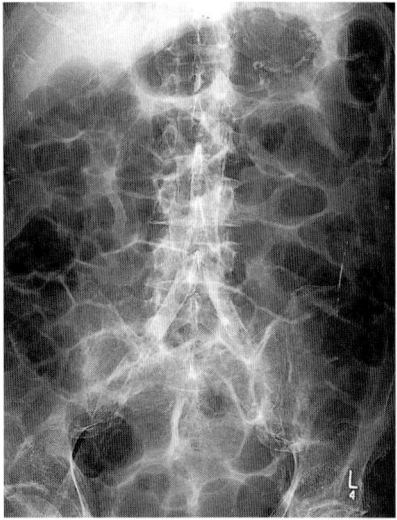

Fig. 3.4 Meteorism. Although there is marked gaseous filling of the bowel, the calibre is normal and there was no cut-off point. (There is also significant vascular calcification.)

Meteorism

identified in other parts of the colon, even when massively distended (**Fig. 3.3**).

The identification of faecal matter in the colon is a reliable discriminating sign between small and large bowel.

This is the name given to the phenomenon of swallowed air seen within the bowel lumen. In adults it can occur secondary to any condition where there is severe pain, and similarly in children, as a sign of distress. It can be difficult to distinguish this radiographic appearance (gas-filled, slightly dilated loops of bowel; **Fig. 3.4**) from intestinal obstruction.

Fat lines

Fat surrounds the abdominal viscera such as the kidneys, spleen, liver, bladder and psoas muscles, and this allows their delineation on x-ray. These fat lines can disappear (which is known as *effacement*) secondary to inflammation, fluid accumulation or displacement by organomegaly.

Absence of the fat lines in normal individuals

1. The outline of the spleen cannot be identified in up to 40% of individuals
2. Loss of a psoas outline occurs in 50% of adults and in 20% of children
3. Loss of fat planes occurs in 20% of individuals.

INTESTINAL OBSTRUCTION

The clinical impression of intestinal obstruction is a frequent indication for requesting an abdominal radiograph. Radiological signs can be elicited which may help to evaluate the level of the obstruction.

Gastric outlet obstruction

The antrum and pyloric regions are the commonest sites of gastric obstruction (**Fig. 3.5**), the most common causes are carcinoma and ulcer. The stomach is usually distended with air and fluid and this is usually best demonstrated on an erect or right lateral decubitus film. Displacement of the adjacent transverse colon by the distended stomach can also be seen. Other causes of gastric dilatation are summarized below.

Other causes of gastric dilatation include:

- Postoperative: vagotomy, especially highly selective vagotomy
- Drugs: opiates and anticholinergics
- Renal failure
- Hypokalaemia
- Heavy metal poisoning.

Duodenal obstruction

In duodenal obstruction, gas and fluid distend the stomach and duodenum.

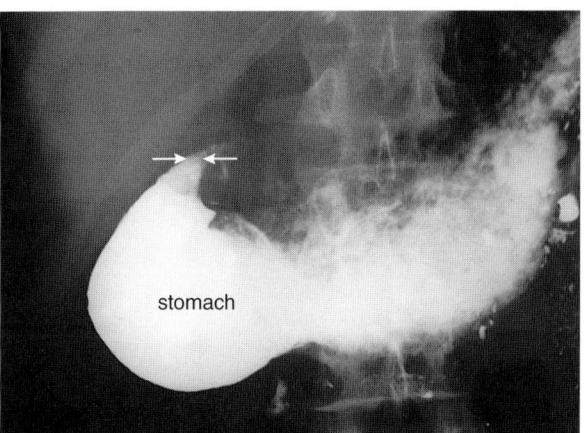

Fig. 3.5 Gastric outlet obstruction.

stomach

Two separate gastric and duodenal air/fluid levels can be seen: the *double bubble sign*.

A left-lateral decubitus projection allows air to enter the dilated duodenum, indicating that the obstruction is distal to the pylorus.

Small bowel obstruction

Note: Small bowel obstruction is usually caused by adhesions, hernias and lesions *outside* the small bowel. Small bowel obstruction is due to adhesions in the majority of cases. Hernias account for 10% (**Fig. 3.6a, b**).

When the small bowel becomes obstructed, accumulation of air and secretions causes dilatation. Normal peristalsis eliminates intestinal contents distal to the level of obstruction, usually within 24 hours.

Abdominal plain films show dilated loops of small bowel, usually measuring more than 3.5 cm in diameter. The degree of small bowel dilatation tends to be greater in patients with true mechanical obstruction than adynamic ileus. As the loops of bowel fill with air, they may assume a 'stepladder' appearance.

Plain film changes may appear after 3–5 hours if there is complete small bowel obstruction, and are usually evident by 12 hours. With incomplete obstruction, the plain x-ray changes may take days to appear. If there is persistent diagnostic difficulty, sequential films are helpful in demonstrating an evolving obstructive pattern. There may be no gas or fluid visible in the small bowel in patients with a high jejunal obstruction.

The *string of beads sign*, due to bubbles of gas trapped between valvulae conniventes on the erect film, results from a dilated small bowel loop filling with fluid. This feature is not normally found in adynamic ileus, and therefore suggests mechanical obstruction.

Suggested imaging protocol for small bowel obstruction

Dedicated small bowel imaging (either small bowel series or enteroclysis) using water-soluble contrast can help delineate the level of the obstruction.

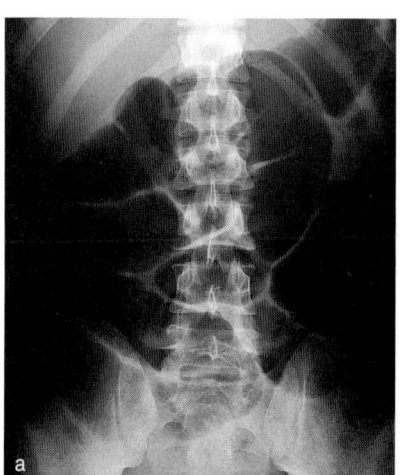 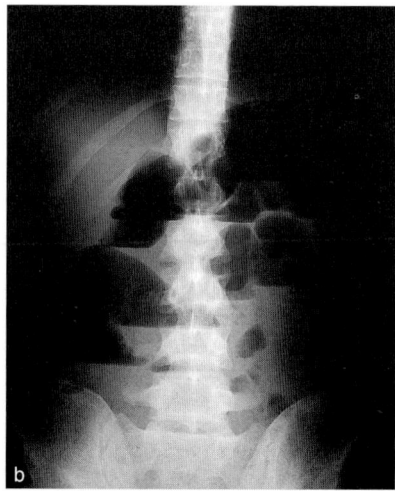

Fig. 3.6 Small bowel obstruction: (**a**) erect and (**b**) supine radiographs. Note the central distribution ('picture in the frame') and the valvulae conniventes.

Large bowel obstruction

Note: Large bowel obstruction is usually caused by adhesions, hernias and lesions *inside* the large bowel (**Fig. 3.7**). Carcinoma is the commonest cause of mechanical large bowel obstruction, with two-thirds of tumours occurring in the sigmoid colon. Diverticulitis is the second commonest cause, with volvulus accounting for only 10% of cases.

Regardless of the site of colonic obstruction, the caecum often shows the most marked distension. When the caecal diameter exceeds 10 cm, the probability of perforation rises sharply.

Obstruction of the left colon is more common than on the right. Small bowel distension may accompany this, if the ileocaecal valve is incompetent (**Fig. 3.7**). When both are distended, appearances may be similar to an ileus. Failure to demonstrate gas in the rectum is therefore an important discriminating feature between true mechanical obstruction and ileus. The finding of rectal gas on the abdominal radiograph suggests that there is not a mechanical obstruction (**Fig. 3.8**).

Suggested imaging protocol in large bowel obstruction

A single-contrast water-soluble enema will confirm obstruction, delineate the level and exclude a pseudo-obstruction.

Small bowel obstruction versus large bowel obstruction

The distinction between small and large bowel obstruction can be difficult. It may be useful to think of the bowel as a picture in a frame: the small bowel being 'the picture' (**Fig. 3.9**) and the colon 'the frame' (**Fig. 3.10**).

The most useful pointers are the size, distribution and mucosal markings of the distended loops. Even with mechanical small bowel obstruction, it is unusual for

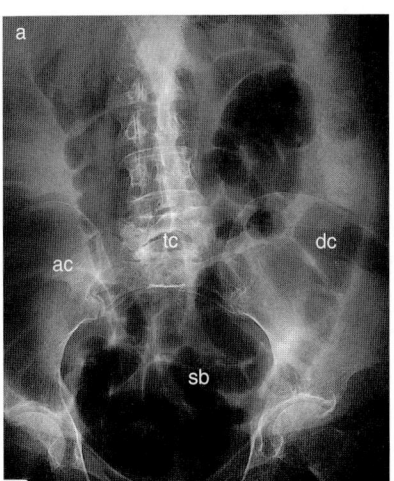
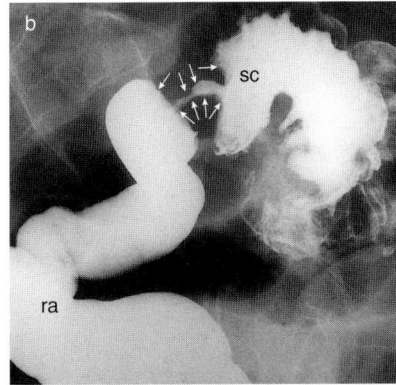

Fig. 3.7 Large bowel obstruction: (**a**) supine radiograph and (**b**) contrast enema. The large bowel is significantly dilated. Note also the prominent small bowel loops indicating an incompetent iliocaecal valve. The underlying lesion was proved to be a sigmoid carcinoma. ac: ascending colon, tc: transverse colon, dc: descending colon, sb: small bowel, ra: rectal ampulla, sc: sigmoid colon, arrows: shouldered edges of sigmoid carcinoma.

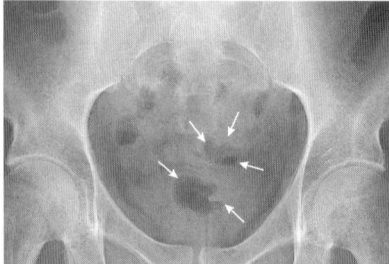

Fig. 3.8 Rectal gas.

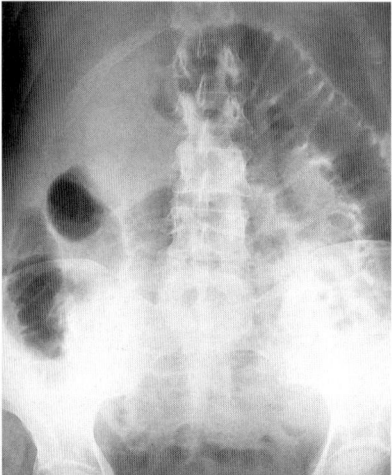

Fig. 3.9 Small bowel obstruction.

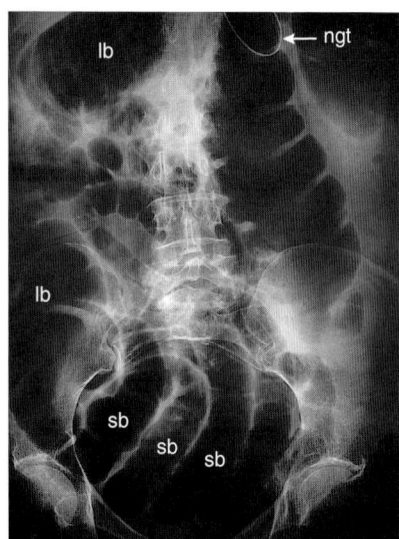

Fig. 3.10 Large bowel (lb) obstruction. Note the valvulae conniventes of the small bowel (sb) indicating iliocaecal valve incompetence. ngt: nasogastric tube.

the bowel diameter to exceed 5 cm. It is also unusual, in large bowel obstruction, for the large bowel diameter to be less than 5 cm. **Table 3.1** summarizes the main features of each type of obstruction.

Contrast examinations of the bowel

Barium remains the mainstay for the radiological evaluation of the small bowel and colon. The small bowel is evaluated using one of two techniques: the small bowel series; or the small bowel enema (also known as *enteroclysis*). In the small bowel series, the patient swallows 200 ml of

barium, and then spot films are taken, usually over 1–2 hours, tracking the progress of the barium through the small bowel and terminal ileum. Apart from the terminal ileum, the small bowel series does not usually include fluoroscopic screening. The small bowel enema (enteroclysis) entails the placing of a nasogastric tube beyond the fourth part of the duodenum and the instillation of 1–2 L of a very dilute suspension of barium. The patient is then screened fluoroscopically, and spot films, usually with compression, are taken of the entire small bowel. Each test has its proponents.

The large bowel is evaluated using the double-contrast barium enema technique. Following appropriate preparation with a low-residue diet and bowel cleansing agent, barium is instilled through a rectal tube (the single-contrast enema; **Fig. 3.11a**). Once the mucosa has been coated, the barium is drained and air

Table 3.1 Radiological signs of small and large bowel obstruction

Radiological feature	Small bowel obstruction	Large bowel obstruction
Location	Central ('picture')	Peripheral ('frame')
Bowel diameter	<5 cm	>5 cm
Valvulae	Present	Absent
Haustra	Absent	Present
Number of loops	Many	Few
Gas in large bowel	No	Yes. Cut-off point

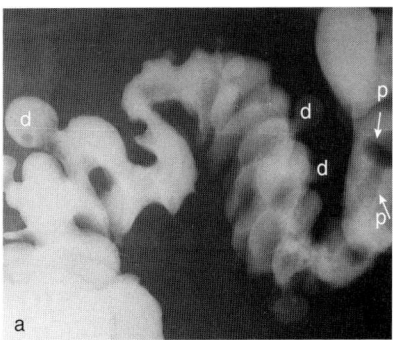 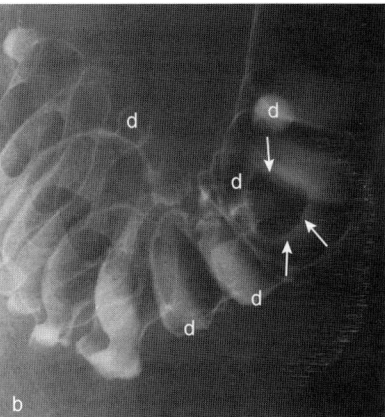

Fig. 3.11 Barium enema: diverticula and 'concealed' polyp (**a**) single and (**b**) double contrast films demonstrate the difference between the diverticulum (d) and the polyp (p). The polyp always appears as a dark 'filling defect' (arrows).

pumped gently into the colon (the double-contrast enema; **Fig. 3.11b**). Standard films are taken in the supine, erect and decubitus positions.

The instant enema

This is performed without bowel preparation, and is designed to show the severity and extent of mucosal disease in ulcerative colitis. It is contraindicated in toxic megacolon and following colonic biopsy.

Water-soluble contrast media

Barium should not be used where there is a risk of intestinal breach or perforation. Barium peritonitis carries with it a significant morbidity and mortality. In this situation, water-soluble contrast media should be employed. There are two commonly used agents: gastrografin (a combination of meglumine diatrizoate and sodium diatrizoate) and niopam (iopamidol). Gastrografin, unlike iopamidol, is hypertonic. Although, therefore, both are safe to use to diagnose a perforation, if gastrografin is aspirated into the bronchi (e.g. during a postgastrectomy upper gastrointestinal examination in an elderly patient) its hypertonicity draws fluid into the airways and can precipitate pulmonary oedema! Because iopamidol is isotonic, this does not occur.

Volvulus

Any segment of bowel with a mesentery can twist to produce a volvulus.

Sigmoid volvulus

This occurs in an elderly population and accounts for three-quarters of colonic volvulus. It is often chronic, sometimes with acute attacks.

Radiological signs of sigmoid volvulus

The obstructed sigmoid loop forms two large compartments that share a double wall, converging at the point of twist. This has been termed the *coffee-bean sign*. The distended sigmoid colonic loop does not usually have prominent haustra. The ahaustral loops of the volvulus can overlap the liver – the *liver overlap sign* – and may also overlap the distended haustral descending colon: the *left flank overlap sign*. The apex of the loop lies high in the abdomen, classically at the level of the tenth thoracic vertebral body, and on the left side. There is more air than fluid in the loop (air:fluid ratio greater than 2:1) than in a caecal volvulus (**Figs 3.12 and 3.13**).

Following a single-contrast enema examination, there is a tapering of the contrast at the point of torsion: the *bird of prey sign* (**Fig. 3.14**).

Caecal volvulus

This occurs when there is malrotation and the caecum has a mesentery. It usually occurs in a younger age group (30–60 years) than sigmoid volvulus.

Radiological signs

In 50% of patients the caecum inverts so that the caecal pole and the appendix lie in the upper left quadrant. This has been termed the *empty caecum* or *comma sign*. In the other 50%, the caecum twists without inversion and still lies on the right side of the abdomen (**Figs 3.15 and 3.16**).

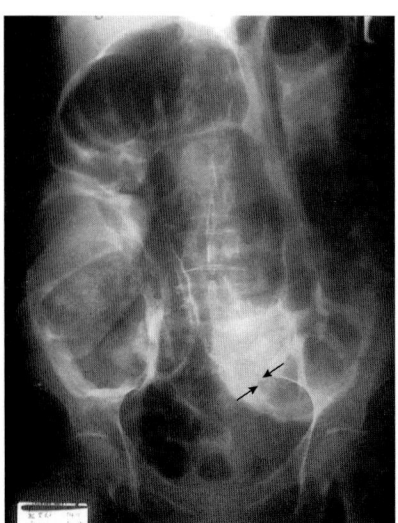

Fig. 3.12 Sigmoid volvulus, supine radiograph. Arrows mark the level of the volvulus.

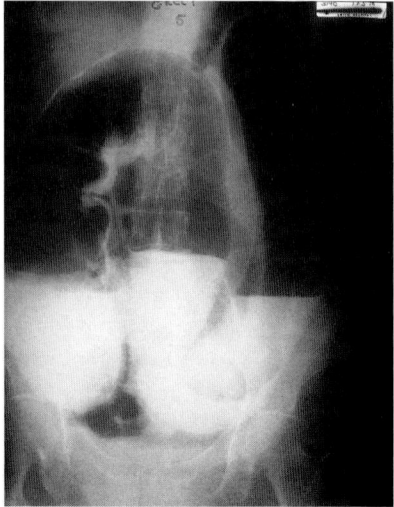

Fig. 3.13 Sigmoid volvulus, erect radiograph.

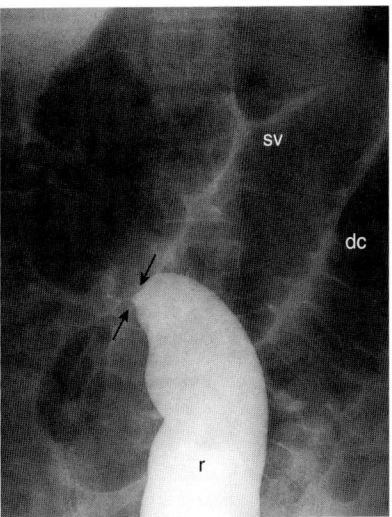

Fig. 3.14 Sigmoid volvulus: the bird of prey sign. Note the sigmoid volvulus (sv) and distended descending colon (dc). r: rectum, →←: point of twisting.

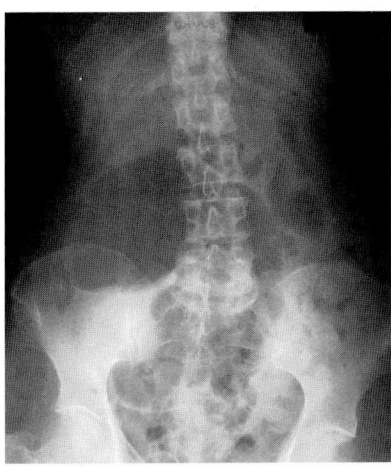

Fig. 3.15 Caecal volvulus, supine radiograph.

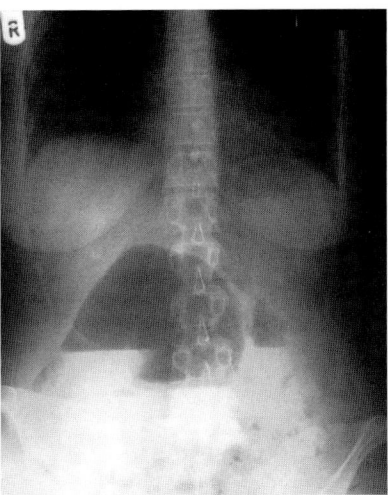

Fig. 3.16 Caecal volvulus, erect radiograph.

Frequently, haustral markings can be seen (compared to sigmoid volvulus whence they are usually absent). There is usually only one large gas and fluid filled bowel loop seen with approximately equal amounts of air and fluid (air:fluid ratio of 1:1). Gaseous and fluid distension of the small bowel may also be seen. Predictably, the large bowel distal to the caecum is empty.

ILEUS AND PSEUDO-OBSTRUCTION

Adynamic ileus

Adynamic or paralytic ileus describes bowel dilatation in the absence of mechanical obstruction. There is absent or decreased intestinal peristalsis, which allows swallowed air to accumulate in the dilated small intestine. The diagnostic sensitivity can be increased by correlating the films with the presence or absence of bowel sounds.

Aetiology of adynamic ileus

(**SAGE**)

- **S**epsis/surgery
- **A**bdominal trauma

41

- **G**eneralized peritonitis
- **E**lectrolyte imbalances.

Pseudo-obstruction (Ogilvie's syndrome)

Acute colonic pseudo-obstruction was first described by Ogilvie. The most common clinical presentation is that of acute abdominal distension which usually occurs within 10 days of the onset of the precipitating pathological process. Abdominal radiographs demonstrate marked colonic distension, which is usually confined to the caecum, ascending and transverse colon. Rectal gas is present.

Note: Ten percent of 'intestinal obstructions' are, in fact, pseudo-obstructions. Ten percent of suspected 'pseudo-obstructions' prove to be mechanical obstructions.

PNEUMOPERITONEUM

Pneumoperitoneum, i.e. the presence of free intraabdominal air, is generally an ominous sign. A perforated abdominal viscus is the commonest pathological cause (in the absence of a history of recent surgery).

Causes of pneumoperitoneum

1. Postoperative
2. Perforation of a hollow viscus
3. Breach of the peritoneum, e.g. stab wound
4. Intraperitoneal infection
5. Via the genital tract in females
6. Idiopathic.

Postoperative pneumoperitoneum

The most common cause of pneumoperitoneum is previous surgery, and the air may take up to 3 weeks to resorb. The patient's body habitus influences the persistence of postoperative pneumoperitoneum, and gas takes longer to resorb in thin patients than in obese patients. *Note:* In a child or an obese patient, free air that persists after the third day should be monitored carefully. In the absence of drains, and with the appropriate clinical presentation, this should raise the possibility of a possible anastomotic leak, and a high index of suspicion should be maintained. The key radiological observation is that of free air under the hemidiaphragm *on an erect chest film* (**Fig. 3.17**). This is easier to identify on the right side, as the left-sided gastric air bubble can be mistaken for free air. The normal variant of Chalaiditi's syndrome, i.e. interposed colonic gas-filled loops between hemidiaphragms and the liver or spleen, should be excluded. This is generally possible, as in this syndrome careful inspection of the interposed bowel loops will reveal mucosal markings **(Fig. 3.18a, b)**.

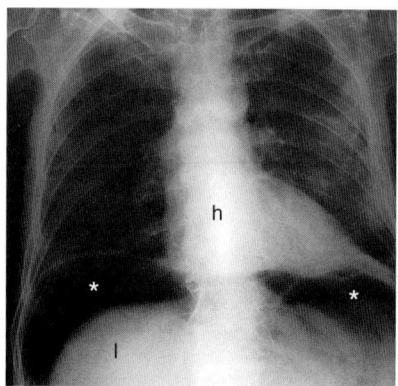

Fig. 3.17 Gross pneumoperitoneum (*) secondary to perforated abdominal viscus. Free air under hemidiaphragm. h: heart, l: liver.

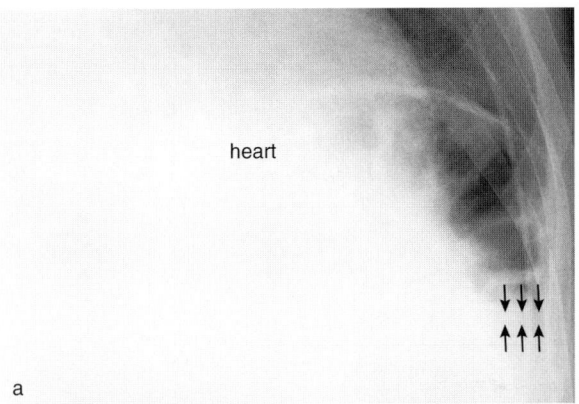

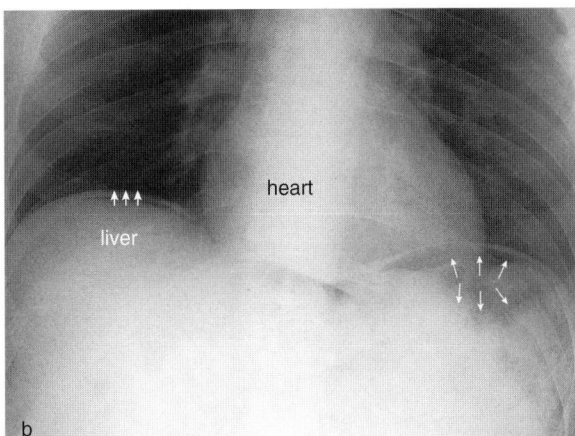

Fig. 3.18(a) Chalaiditi's syndrome: erect chest radiograph. Note the gas shadows under the left hemi-diaphragm. The normal mucosal pattern is clearly identified however, so perforation is excluded. **(b)** A perforation. Here there is free air under the left hemidiaphragm. (The diagnosis was a perforated duodenal ulcer.) Arrows: pneumoperitoneum.

Signs of intraperitoneal air on supine films

There are a number of radiological signs described which can help identify the presence of intraperitoneal air on a supine film. It is imperative that the clinician has a knowledge of these, as it is not uncommon to be faced with very ill patients who may not be fit enough to undergo erect or even decubitus examinations.

Rigler's sign

Rigler's sign describes the sharp delineation of the bowel wall on plain radiographs, and is caused by the presence of air adjacent to both the mucosa and serosa (**Fig. 3.19**).

Falciform ligament sign

Free air delineates the falx and this appears as a sickle-shaped density in the right upper quadrant which extends from the liver to the umbilicus (**Fig. 3.19**).

Inverted V sign

This sign is due to the surrounding of the lateral umbilical ligaments by air. It is identified as two lines extending from the midpoint of each inguinal ligament to the umbilicus (**Fig. 3.20**).

Football or dome sign

Air forms an ellipse over free fluid in the upper abdomen.

43

Urachus sign

The urachus is the remnant of the allantois. The free air outlines both sides of this

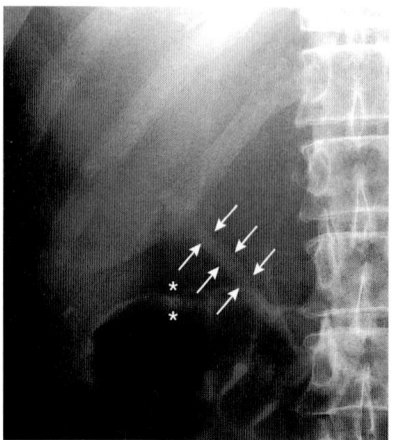

Fig. 3.19 The falciform ligament sign (arrows) and Rigler's sign (*).

midline structure between the pelvis and the umbilicus.

Parahepatic air sign

A circular opacity over the anterior inferior border of the liver.

Morrison's pouch sign

Free air trapped in Morrison's pouch.

Triangle sign

Free air between three loops of bowel.

Scrotal air sign

Air fills the scrotum via the processus vaginalis.

Cupola sign

Air trapped below the central tendon of the diaphragm.

Fig. 3.20 Inverted V sign.

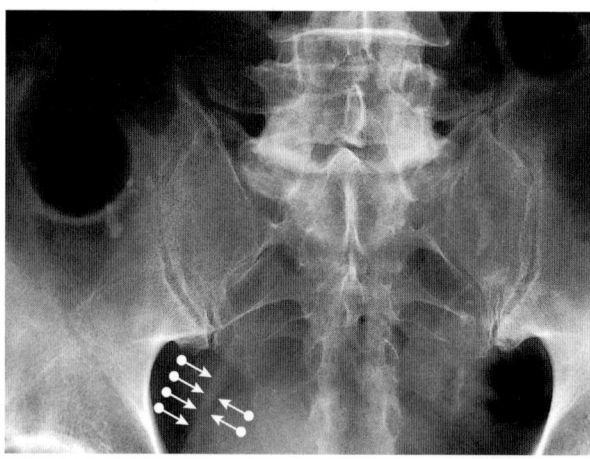

SEPSIS

Appendicitis

Although acute appendicitis remains a clinical diagnosis, plain radiographs can reveal abnormalities in up to 50% of patients (**Figs 3.21 and 3.22**). A summary of radiographic findings is given below.

Radiographic findings in acute appendicitis

1. Appendicolith (**Fig. 3.21**)

(a) Present in up to 14% of patients with appendicitis

(b) Usually bigger than a faecolith

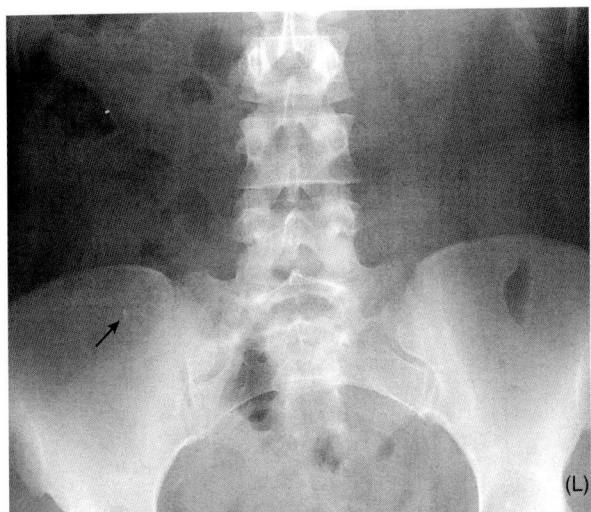

Fig. 3.21 Plain film showing appendicolith (arrow). Diagnosis was confirmed at laparotomy.

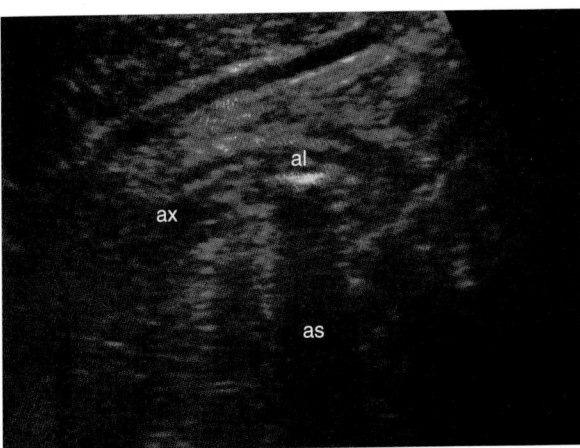

Fig. 3.22 Ultrasound showing appendicolith (al). ax: vermiform appendix, as: acoustic shadowing.

(c) Often have a radiolucent centre

(d) 50% of symptomatic patients with an identifiable appendicolith have developed perforation.

2. Appendiceal masses (**Fig. 3.23**).

(a) May produce mass effect

(b) Displace adjacent bowel loops.

Subphrenic and subhepatic abscess

In the plain film evaluation of a right subphrenic abscess, the eleventh rib (the level of the triangular ligament) provides a useful landmark. Subphrenic collections tend to produce abnormal gas

45

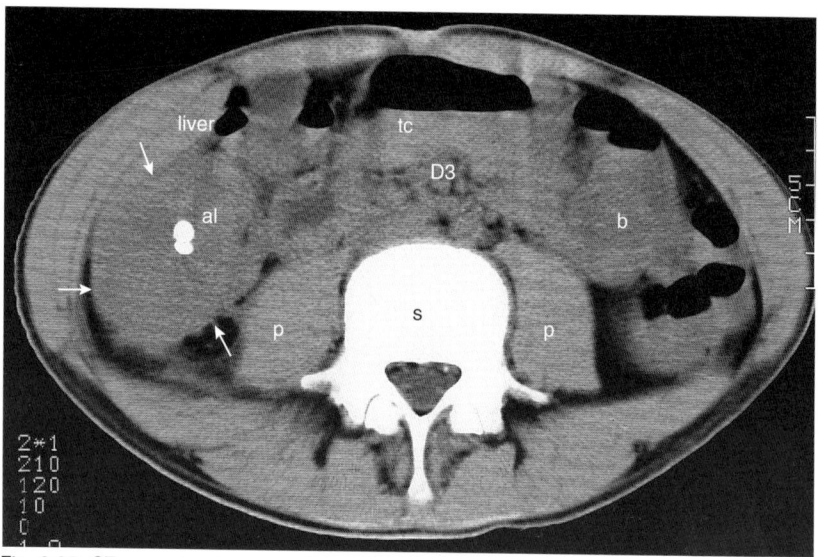

Fig. 3.23 CT scan showing appendiceal mass (arrows). b: bowel, al: appendicolith, p: psoas, s: spine, D3: third part of duodenum, tc: transverse colon.

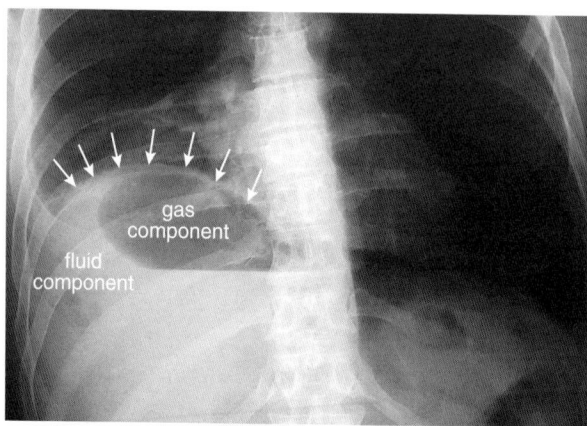

Fig. 3.24 Erect chest radiograph: right subphrenic abscess. The abscess has both a gas and a fluid component. Note the prominent fluid level (arrows indicate diaphragm).

collections above the eleventh rib (**Fig. 3.24**).

An abscess in the right anterior subhepatic space displaces the transverse colon inferiorly. A mass in the posterior subhepatic space (Morrison's pouch) displaces the duodenum inferiorly, medially and posteriorly.

Left subphrenic abscesses usually remain localized and are unlikely to pass beyond the phrenicocolic ligament. The diagnosis of abscess is usually confirmed on ultrasound or CT (**Fig. 3.25a, b**) and both techniques allow intervention and drainage.

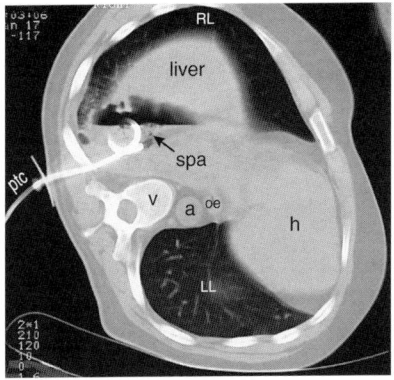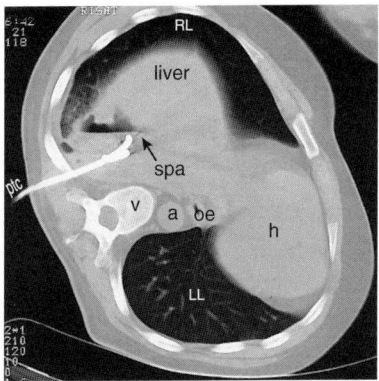

Fig. 3.25 CT of subphrenic abscess (spa) (**a**) during and (**b**) immediately following drainage. The patient is in the decubitus position. The abscess is identified and a pigtail drain (ptc) is placed percutaneously into the collection. Twenty minutes later there has been a significant reduction in the volume. RL: right lung, LL: left lung, v: vertebra, oe: oesophagus, a: aorta, h: heart.

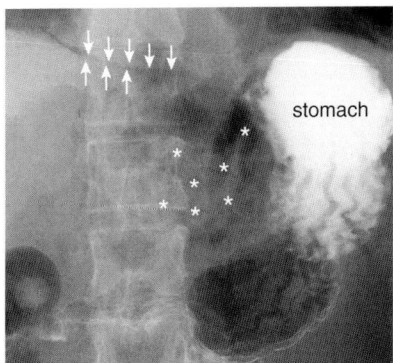

Fig. 3.26 Retroperitoneal perforation. Water-soluble upper gastrointestinal series. Note the 'bubble-wrap' appearance (*) of the retroperitoneal perforation adjacent to the lesser curve of the stomach. There is also an intraperitoneal component, seen as free air under the diaphragm (arrows).

Retroperitoneal abscesses

In retroperitoneal duodenal perforation, plain films demonstrate an abnormality in one-third of cases. The tear is usually at the junction of the second and third parts, and will be delineated with water-soluble contrast. The pattern of extraduodenal gas is distinctive and looks a little like commercial bubble-wrap (**Fig. 3.26**).

In retroperitoneal colonic perforation, plain radiographs often show a retrocolic mass and gas collection. The ipsilateral psoas muscle may be obscured by the soft tissue density, but the properitoneal fat plane is usually intact.

Acute diverticulitis

Fifteen percent of patients with diverticulosis will develop diverticulitis. Of those that subsequently perforate, 75% will occur into the retroperitoneum. This may lead to subacute symptoms, delaying the diagnosis. Retroperitoneal perforation causes local inflammation, limiting the volume of escaping colonic effluent. Although the diagnosis of diverticulosis is usually made on barium studies (**Fig. 3.27**), CT and MRI are also sensitive in identifying the diverticula (**Fig. 3.28**).

Peridiverticular collections may be identified as extracolonic air/fluid levels during contrast examinations. It is important to note that if there is any clinical suspicion of diverticular perforation, the examination should be performed with a water-soluble contrast (**Fig. 3.29; p. 49**).

Ischaemic colitis

Any part of the large bowel may be affected but (in descending order) the splenic flexure, descending colon and terminal ileum are the comonest sites.

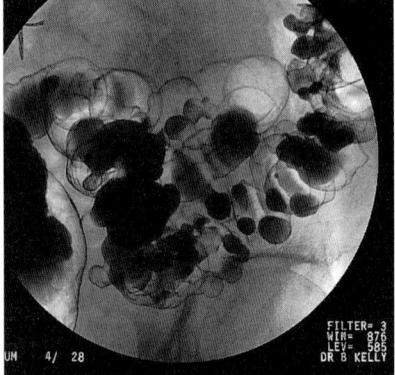

Fig. 3.27 Diverticular disease on barium enema.

Non-gangrenous form

The plain radiographs may be normal, or may show mild large bowel dilatation, a gasless abdomen, or luminal narrowing with *thumbprinting* (**Fig. 3.30a**). An instant enema (i.e. one performed without prior bowel prepartion) will confirm the diagnosis. If perforation is suspected, barium should never be introduced. A water-soluble contrast medium (e.g. gastrografin or iopamidol) should be substituted (**Fig. 3.30b**).

Typical changes of acute ischaemic colitis on instant enema include (**Fig. 3.30b**)

- Narrowing of the affected bowel
- Thumbprinting
- Funnelling of the bowel over a short segment at the transition from normal to abnormal bowel.

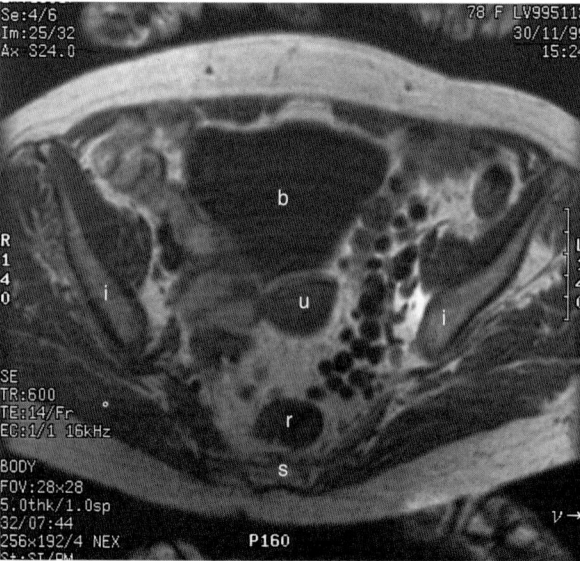

Fig. 3.28 Diverticular disease on MRI. b: bladder, u: uterus, i: ilium, r: rectum, s: sacrum.

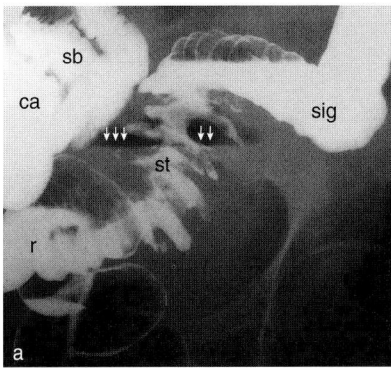
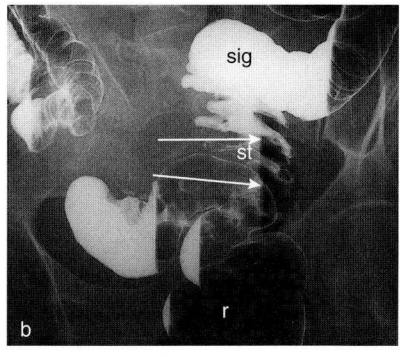

Fig. 3.29 Peridiverticular collection, erect and decubitus films, contrast enema. (**a**) There is a stricture in the sigmoid colon (sig). In addition there is an extracolonic fluid collection behind the sigmoid colon: note the air/fluid level (short arrows). (**b**) The decubitus film confirms the collection (long arrows). r: rectum, st: stricture, sb: small bowel, ca: caecum.

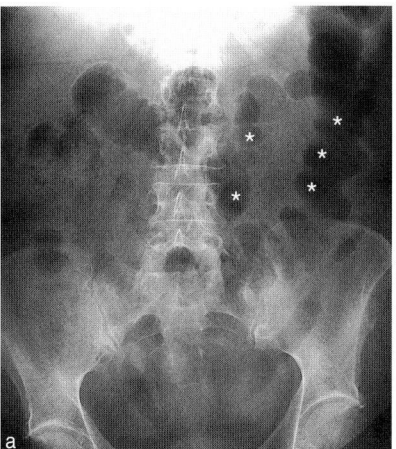
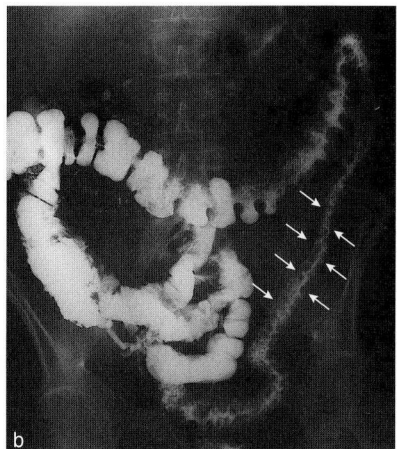

Fig. 3.30 Ischaemic colitis: (**a**) plain abdominal radiograph and (**b**) water-soluble contrast enema. Note the gross mucosal irregularity following water-soluble enema. (*Thumbprinting, left colon.)

A double-contrast enema should be performed 4–8 weeks after the acute attack has resolved. If a stricture has formed it is usually symmetrical except where pseudo-diverticula have developed. Persistence of thumbprinting for longer than 10 days is associated with stricture formation. These strictures tend to be long and tapered but shorter than the original ischaemic segment (**Fig. 3.31a, b**).

Gangrenous form

Toxic megacolon (vide infra) can develop in gangrenous ischaemic colitis. Additional radiological features include intramural gas, either from disintegration of the bowel wall or clostridium contamination, free perforation, or gas extending into the portal vein.

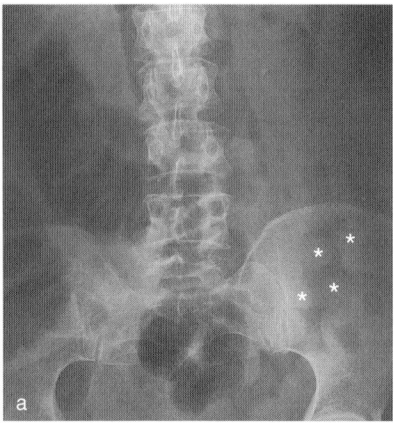 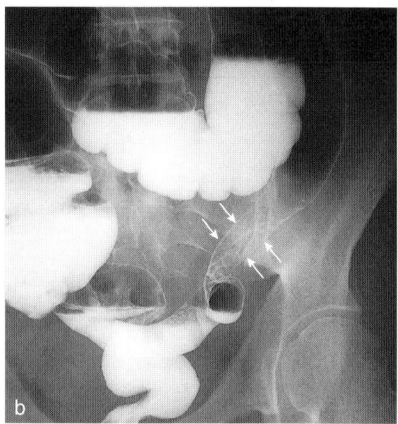

Fig. 3.31 Ischaemic colitis: (**a**) plain abdominal radiograph. There is gross thumbprinting of the left colon (*). (**b**) Barium enema, 8 weeks later. Note the smooth, tapering stricture.

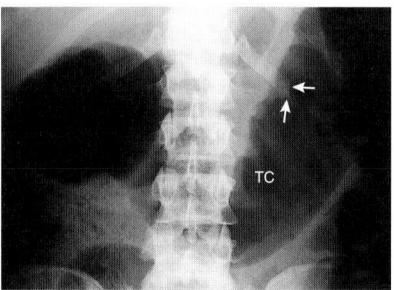

Fig. 3.32 Toxic megacolon: abdominal radiograph. The transverse diameter of the transverse colon (TC) is significantly enlarged. Note thumbprinting of the mucosa (arrows). (The diagnosis was ulcerative colitis.)

Toxic megacolon

Fifteen percent of patients with ulcerative colitis have acute symptoms. The most severe manifestation is toxic megacolon, which occurs in 2%. A gas-distended colon with a transverse diameter of greater than 6.5 cm should be viewed with suspicion (**Fig. 3.32**). Other plain-film findings include mucosal thickening and thumbprinting. A barium enema should never be requested when the diagnosis of toxic megacolon is suspected.

Further Reading

Margulis A R, Burhenne H J 1993 Practical alimentary tract radiology. St Louis: Mosby Year Book.

4 Imaging in Hepatobiliary Disease

> **Topics included in this chapter**
> - The gallbladder
> - The biliary tree
> - The pancreas
> - Focal liver lesions

The diagnosis in hepatopancreaticobiliary pathology is generally made on cross-sectional imaging. However, the plain radiograph can be invaluable in the preliminary evaluation of many conditions. Ultrasound usage is becoming more widespread among clinicians, and therefore a brief outline of common ultrasonic appearances is given. Mention is also made of percutaneous transhepatic cholangiography (PTC) and endoscopic retrograde cholangiopancreatography (ERCP).

THE GALLBLADDER

Gallstones

Abdominal radiograph

The proportion of gallstones visible on plain films is between 20% and 30%. These are seen typically as laminated densities in the right upper quadrant of the abdomen (**Fig. 4.1**).

Occasionally, stellate lucencies are seen in the region of the gallbladder. These reflect gaseous fissures within the calculi. The pattern of the radiolucency is triradiate, and for this reason is known as the *Mercedes Benz* (or *Isle of Man*) *sign* (**Fig. 4.2**).

Ultrasound

Ultrasound is the method of choice in detecting gallstones, with a sensitivity of 98%. Gallstones appear as echogenic (bright) lesions which cast a strong posterior (black) shadow distally: the so-called *acoustic shadow*. It is of central importance to appreciate that ultrasound waves cannot

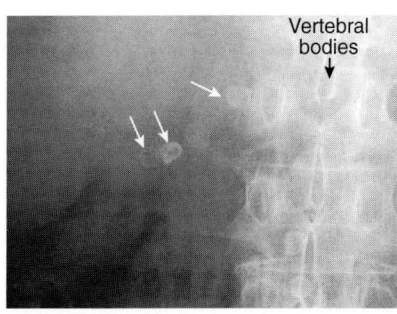

Fig. 4.1 Typical appearance of laminated gallstones (arrows): plain abdominal radiograph.

penetrate either gas, bone or calcified structures. When the beam impinges on these, it is immediately reflected off their surface. Because no sound waves penetrate the rest of the structure, there is a dark band behind the surface: this band is the acoustic shadow (**Fig. 4.3**).

Small polyps are not infrequently detected within the gallbladder on ultrasound. These may be indistinguishable from stones, except that there is no posterior acoustic shadowing (**Fig. 4.4**).

Ultrasound can also detect the presence of layered echogenic bile within the gallbladder. This has been associated with cholecystitis, extrahepatic biliary obstruction and prolonged fasting. The echoes are formed by pigment granules composed of calcium bilirubinate.

The gallbladder wall thickness can reliably be measured by ultrasound and usually is 2–3 mm in diameter. In acute cholecystitis, the wall becomes thicker and has a dark halo around it. Enhanced CT demonstrates the inflamed wall as a bright enhancing ring (**Fig. 4.5**).

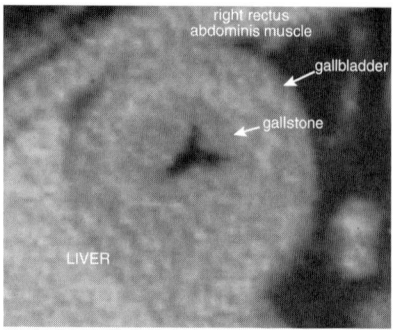

Fig. 4.2 CT image of Mercedes Benz sign.

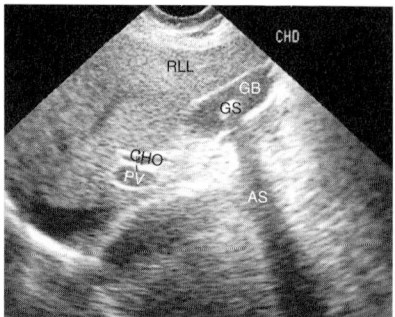

Fig. 4.3 Ultrasound of gallbladder (GB) demonstrating the typical appearance of a gallstone (GS). RLL: right lobe liver, AS: acoustic shadowing, CHD: common hepatic duct, PV: portal vein.

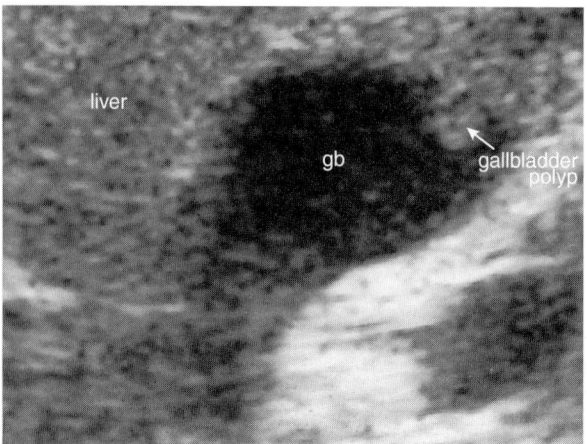

Fig. 4.4 Gallbladder polyp. Note the absence of posterior acoustic shadowing. gb: gall bladder.

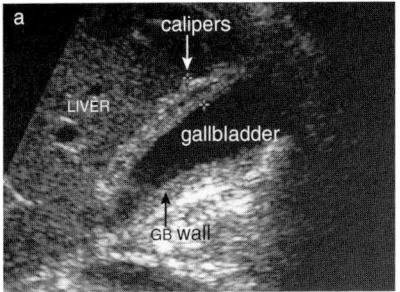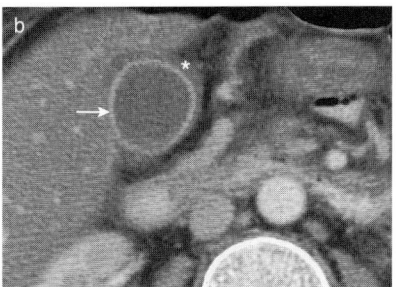

Fig. 4.5 Thickened gallbladder wall in acute cholecystitis. (**a**) Ultrasonic appearance: calipers placed on the gallbladder wall measure the wall thickness at 8.1 mm (normal thickness 2 mm). (**b**) CT appearance: intense ring of enhancement within the gallbladder wall (arrow) surrounded by oedema (*).

Occasionally the gallbladder is so shrunken by chronic cholecystitis that only a dense band is appreciated on ultrasound. This is known as a *wall echo shadow* or WES gallbladder (**Fig. 4.6**).

Other gallbladder pathology: abdominal radiograph

Porcelain gallbladder

This occurs in chronic cholecystitis and is seen as a rim of calcification around the gallbladder. The condition has a high association with gallbladder carcinoma (**Fig. 4.7**).

Limey bile

In chronic cholecystitis the bile can become thickened and *layering out* or sedimentation can occur. Concentrations of calcium can accumulate within the sediment, allowing this layer of calcium to be seen on the abdominal radiograph or CT. This is known as *limey bile* (**Fig. 4.8**).

Gallstone ileus

This occurs when a gallstone erodes into the small bowel and impacts in the distal

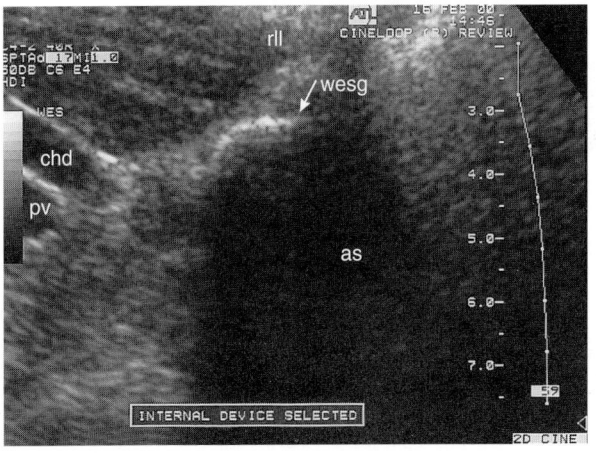

Fig. 4.6 Ultrasound of WES gallbladder. wesg: wall echo shadow gallbladder, rll: right lobe of liver, chd: common hepatic duct, pv: portal vein, as: acoustic shadow.

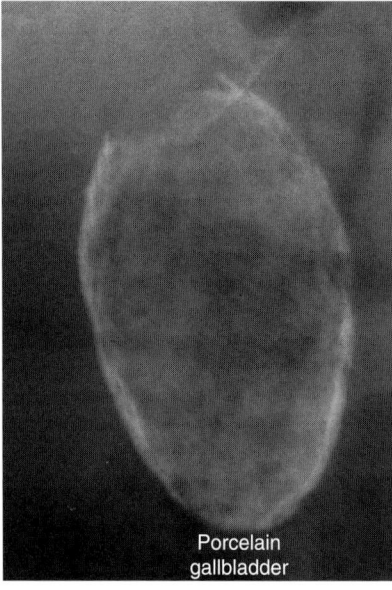

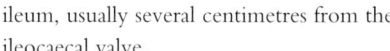
Porcelain
gallbladder

Fig. 4.7 Porcelain gallbladder: plain
abdominal radiograph.

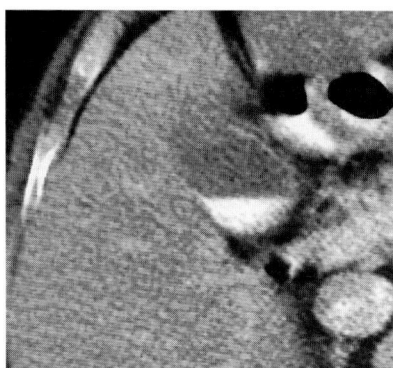

Fig. 4.8 Limey bile: CT image.

ileum, usually several centimetres from the
ileocaecal valve.

Radiographic features of gallstone ileus
(**Fig. 4.9**)

- Gas in the biliary tree
- Gallstone in an abnormal position
  (usually right iliac fossa)
- Small bowel obstruction.

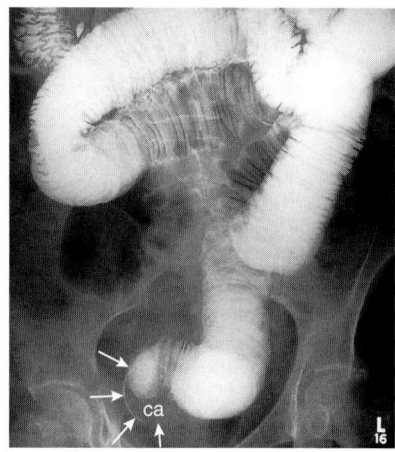

Fig. 4.9 Gallstone ileus. There are distended loops of barium-filled small
bowel. The calculus (ca) is seen as a filling
defect in the right fossa (arrows).

THE BILIARY TREE

Abdominal radiograph

Gas can be identified on the abdominal
radiograph, within the biliary tree, following endoscopic retrograde cholangiopancreatography (ERCP), sphincterotomy and
choledochoenteric surgery. In the absence
of recent intervention or manipulation, the
presence of gas within the biliary tree may

signal cholangitis. Gas is demonstrated as a
dark branching pattern within the liver
(**Figs 4.10 and 4.11**). The important differential diagnosis is that of portal vein air.
This latter sign, which is associated with
pathological conditions and is ominous in
adults, extends more peripherally (within
2 cm of the capsule) than biliary gas.

Ultrasound of the biliary tree

The common hepatic duct normally measures less than 6 mm. It is identified as a small, slim tube sitting on top of the larger portal vein (**Fig. 4.12**).

Ultrasound has a high level of accuracy in predicting the level and the cause of biliary obstruction. Up to 80% of bile duct stones can be identified with ultrasound (**Fig. 4.13**). CT can also identify biliary dilatation and an obstructing calculus (**Figs 4.14 and 4.15**).

Similarly, the left and right bile ducts sit anterior to their respective portal vein branches. These ducts typically measure 1–3 mm in diameter. In patients with an extrahepatic cause of jaundice (e.g. carcinoma of the pancreas), both the intrahepatic ducts *and* the extrahepatic common duct should be dilated. In patients with an intrahepatic cause (e.g. a tumour at the porta hepatis) only the intrahepatic ducts should be dilated (**Fig. 4.16**).

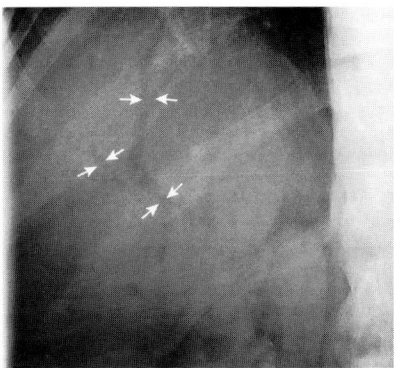

Fig. 4.10 Intrabiliary air: plain abdominal radiograph. Air appears as a dark branching pattern within the liver (arrows).

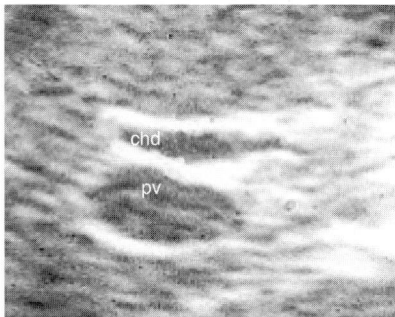

Fig. 4.12 Ultrasound of the normal porta hepatis: cholelithiasis. chd: common hepatic duct, pv: portal vein.

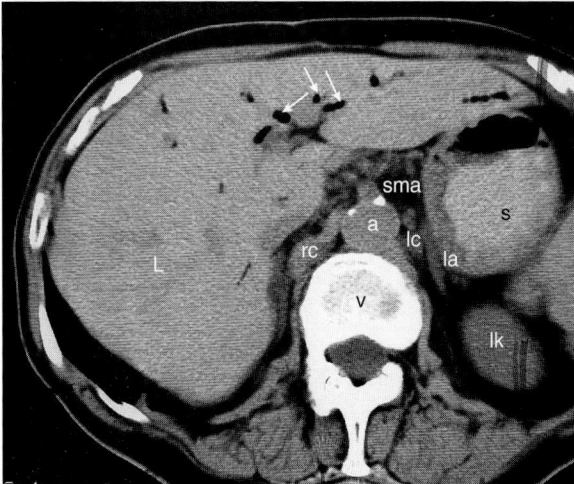

Fig. 4.11 Intrabiliary air: CT appearance. The air is seen as a very dark branching pattern within the liver (L) (arrows). sma: superior mesenteric artery, a: aorta, rc: right crus of diaphragm, lc: left crus of diaphgram, s: stomach, la: left adrenal gland, lk: left kidney.

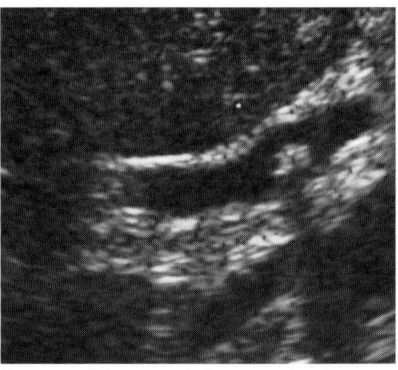
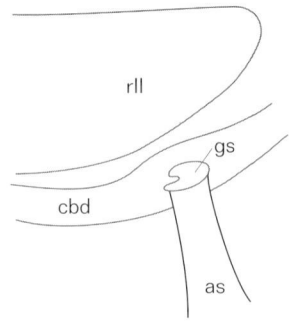

Fig. 4.13 Ultrasound showing dilated common bile duct with stone at the lower end. RLL: right lobe of liver, cbd: common bile duct, gs: gallstone, as: acoustic shadowing.

Percutaneous transhepatic cholangiography

Percutaneous transhepatic cholangiography (PTC) involves the percutaneous placement of a small (20–22 G) needle into a bile duct, typically under fluoroscopy. Currently 98% of dilated ducts and 80% of undiluted ducts can be punctured. Once punctured, the duct is opacified by the slow injection of contrast. Hence it is possible to track the progress of the contrast down the duct system into the duodenum and identify the level of an obstruction (**Fig 4.17a, b**).

The strength of this technique is that it provides a mechanism for intervention within the biliary tree. This has been especially useful in the palliation of malignant disease, with the percutaneous placement of stents and drains to relieve obstructive jaundice (**Fig. 4.18**). The technique has a complication rate of 2% and a mortality rate of 1%. It should be seen as complimentary to ERCP and is more useful than the former in identifying (and treating) diseases at or above the porta.

Endoscopic retrograde cholangiopancreatography

Like PTC, ERCP has the capability to opacify and intervene within the biliary tree. A particular advantage is its ability to biopsy abnormal-looking areas. It is better than PTC in dealing with lesions at the lower end of the bile duct, e.g. retained gallstones (**Fig. 4.19;** p. 58), post-cholecystectomy. It has a morbidity rate of less than 3% and a mortality rate of 0.2%, due mainly to pancreatitis, or septicaemia following cholangitis.

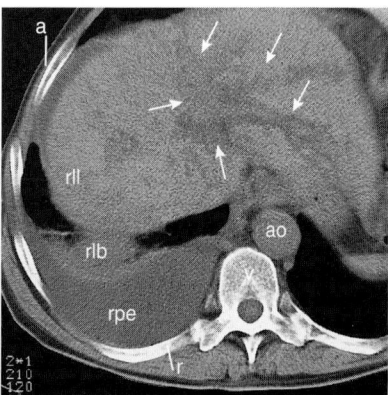

Fig. 4.14 CT demonstrating biliary dilatation (arrows). ao: aorta, rpe: right pleural infusion, rlb: right lung base, rll: right lobe liver, v: vertebral body, a: anterior abdominal wall.

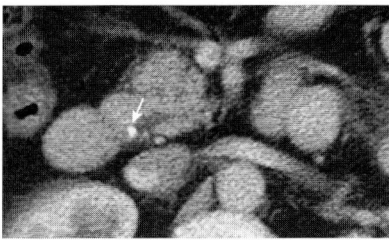 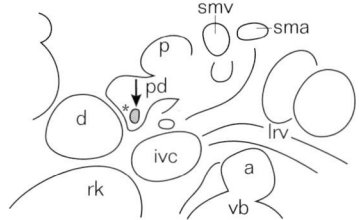

Fig. 4.15 CT of the biliary tree showing calculus (arrowed) at the lower end of the common bile duct. p: pancreas, smv: superior mesenteric vein, sma: superior mesenteric artery, pd: pancreatic duct, d: duodenum, ivc: inferior vena cava, lrv: left renal view, rk: right kidney, a: aorta, vb: vertebral body.

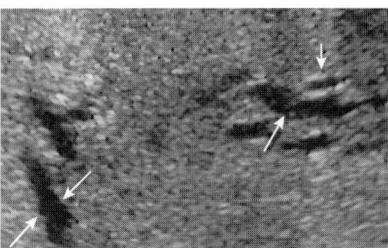 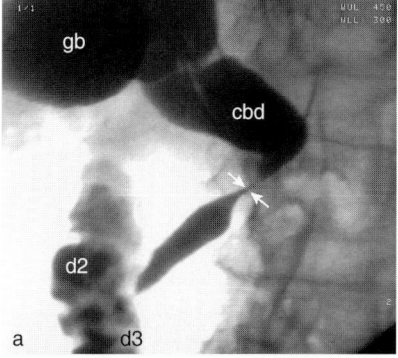

Fig. 4.16 Ultrasound showing intrahepatic duct dilatation. The double-duct sign, i.e. portal vein (short arrow) and bile ducts (long arrow).

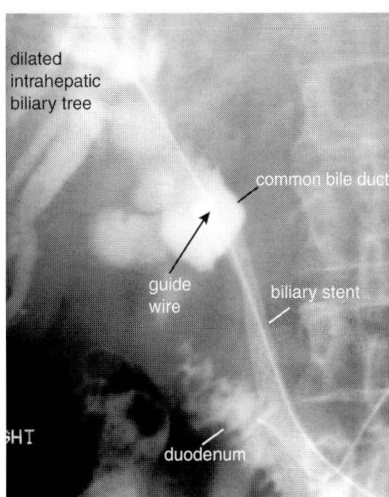 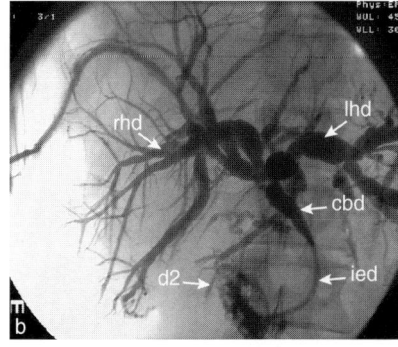

Fig. 4.18 Biliary stent placement. The biliary tree is massively distended. The stent is in position between the common bile duct and the duodenum.

Fig. 4.17 PTC. a Cholangiocarcinoma (arrows). b The internal–external drain passed through it to relieve the obstruction. gb: gallbladder, cbd: common bile duct, d2: second part of duodenum, d3: third part of duodenum, rhd: right hepatic duct, lhd: left hepatic duct, ied: internal external drain.

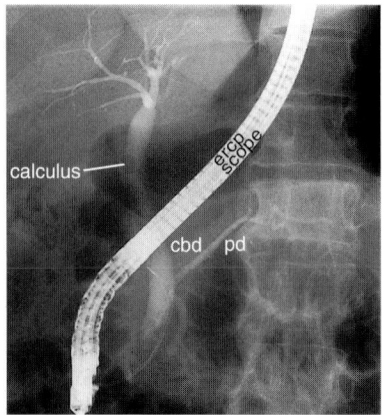

Fig. 4.19 ERCP showing calculus at the mid common bile duct (cbd). pd: pancreatic duct.

Magnetic resonance cholangiopancreatography

The role of magnetic resonance cholangiopancreatography (MRCP) is currently being evaluated, but its use to date suggests that it may have a very significant part to play in the evaluation of the biliary tree (**Figs 4.20–4.24**). Unlike PTC and ERCP it is non-invasive and has no ionizing radiation associated with it.

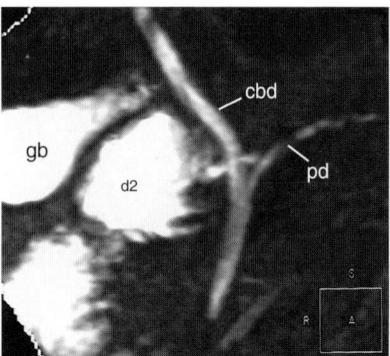

Fig. 4.20 Normal biliary tree: MRI. gb: gallbladder, cbd: common bile duct, pd: pancreatic duct, d2: second part of duodenum.

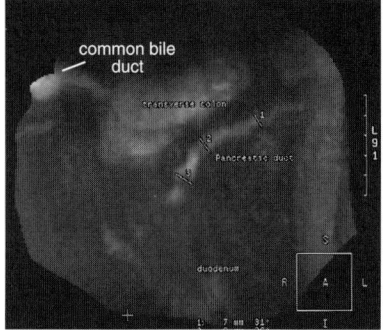

Fig. 4.22 Dilated pancreatic duct: MRI. Measurements: 1 = 7 mm, 2 = 9 mm, 3 = 10 mm (normal pancreatic duct measurement < 3 mm).

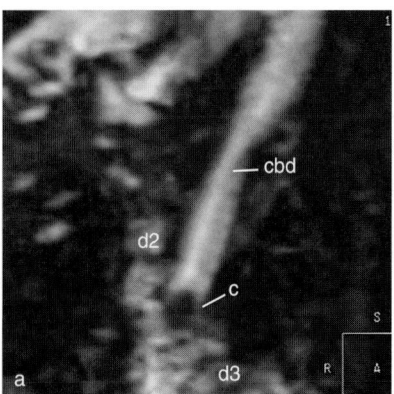

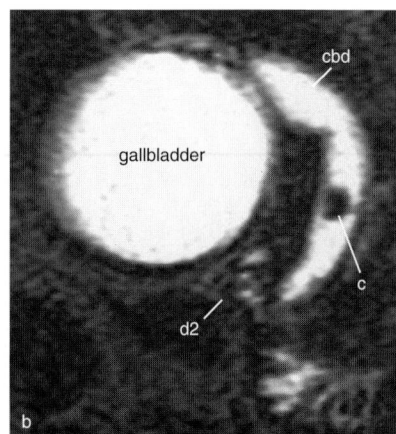

Fig. 4.21a and **b** Calculus (c) in the common bile duct (cbd): MRI. d2: second part of duodenum, d3: third part of duodenum.

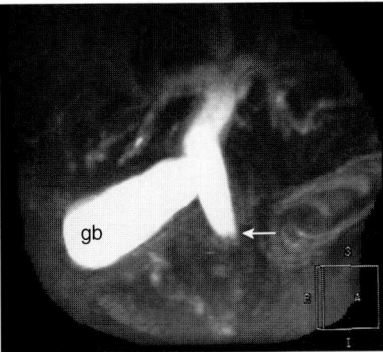

Fig. 4.23 Cholangiocarcinoma: MRI. The gallbladder (gb) is distended, as is the common bile duct. Note also the sudden occlusion of the distal duct (arrow) by the cholangiocarcinoma.

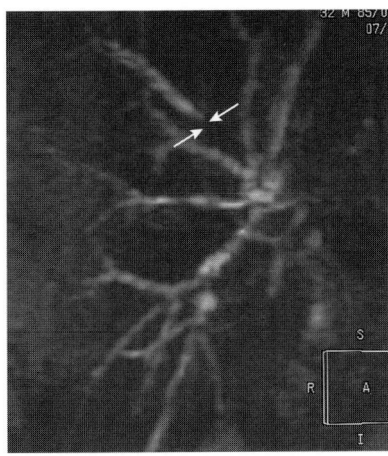

Fig. 4.24 Sclerosing cholangitis: MRI. Note the classical 'beading' of the hepatic duct system.

THE PANCREAS

Pancreatitis

Radiological assessment of the pancreas in pancreatitis is generally performed using cross-sectional techniques, in particular computed tomography (CT). However, specific radiological features of pancreatitis have been described on the plain abdominal radiograph. These include the *sentinel loop sign*, caused by a ileus of the duodenum or localised adjacent small bowel loops, and the *colon cut-off sign*, also known as *Stuart's sign* (**Fig. 4.25**). This latter sign refers to an abrupt change in the calibre of the transverse colon in the area overlying the pancreas.

In addition, acute pancreatitis is usually accompanied by pleural effusions, typically left sided, and basal atelectasis, both of which are visible on the chest radiograph.

On ultrasound, the pancreas is diffusely swollen, but in a significant proportion of cases it may be obscured by overlying bowel gas. A CT scan is usually diagnostic (**Fig. 4.26**), demonstrating gland enlarge-ment and inflammatory changes in the surrounding fat planes.

CT is the imaging method of choice for the surveillance of patients with complex pancreatitis. Cross-sectional imaging allows the delineation of pancreatic necrotic foci (**Fig. 4.27**), inflammatory pancreatic masses, and fluid collections (**Fig. 4.28 and 4.29**; p. 61).

Pancreatic carcinoma

Pancreatic carcinoma has a very poor prognosis. The radiological diagnosis remains challenging, and relies heavily on cross-sectional imaging. The focal lesion generally appears darker than the surrounding parenchyma, both on ultrasound and CT. This is not a specific appearance, and a focal area of pancreatitis can be identical (**Fig. 4.30**; p. 61). CT allows preoperative staging of the tumour, and can help eliminate those patients (80–90%) for whom surgical resection is not possible.

CT signs of pancreatic carcinoma

- Focal low–attenuation lesion.
- A disproportionate sized area within the pancreas. (The pancreas normally atrophies with age, and therefore focal enlarged areas must be viewed with suspicion.)
- Enlargement of the pancreatic duct (normally less than 3 mm), especially when combined with common bile duct dilatation (normally less than 6 mm). This association is called the *double-duct sign*.
- Loss of the perivascular mesenteric fat plane.*

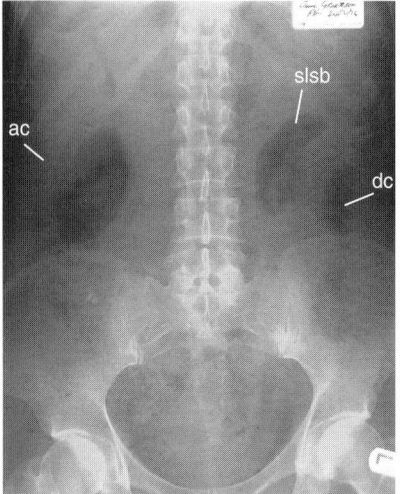

Fig. 4.25 Stuart's sign. slsb: sentinel loop of small bowel, ac: ascending colon, dc: descending colon.

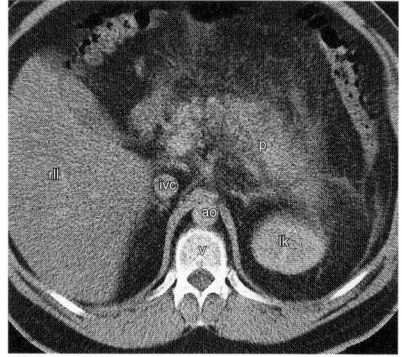

Fig. 4.26 CT scan showing pancreatitis (see fig. 4.27 for caption details).

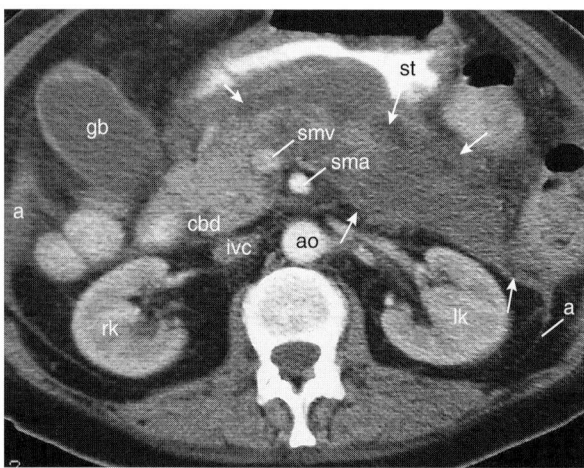

Fig. 4.27 Contrast-enhanced CT scan showing pancreatitis. The pancreas (arrows) is diffusely enlarged. Note the darker area of necrosis and fluid within it. The superior mesenteric artery (sma) is seen behind the body. The normal cuff of fat around it helps to differentiate inflammation from malignancy (where it may be absent). The finding of inflammatory changes and ascites (a) in the anterior pararenal planes bilaterally is characteristic. p: pancreas, gb: gallbladder, ao: aorta, ivc: inferior vena cava, cbd: common bile duct, smv: superior mesenteric vein, st: stomach, lk: left kidney, rk: right kidney.

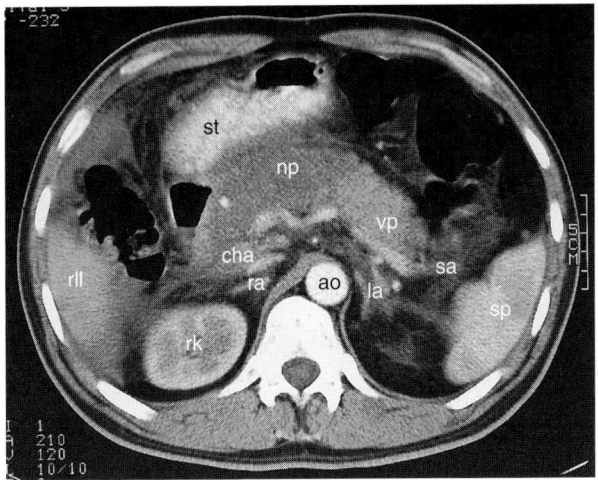

Fig. 4.28 Contrast-enhanced CT demonstrating pancreatic necrosis. st: stomach, np: necrotic pancreas, vp: viable pancreas, cha: common hepatic artery, sa: splenic artery, ra: right adrenal, la: left adrenal, ao: aorta, rll: right lobe of liver, rk: right kidney, sp: spleen.

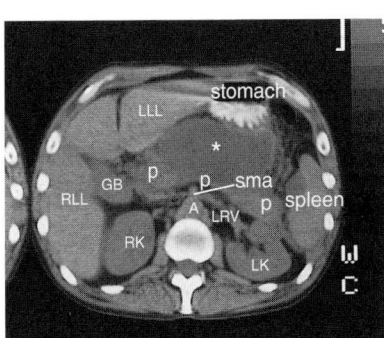

Fig. 4.29 CT scan demonstrating pancreatic pseudocyst (*). LLL: left lobe of liver, RLL: right lobe of liver, GB: gallbladder, p: pancreas, RK: right kidney, LK: left kidney, SMA: superior mesenteric artery, LRV: left renal vein, A: aorta.

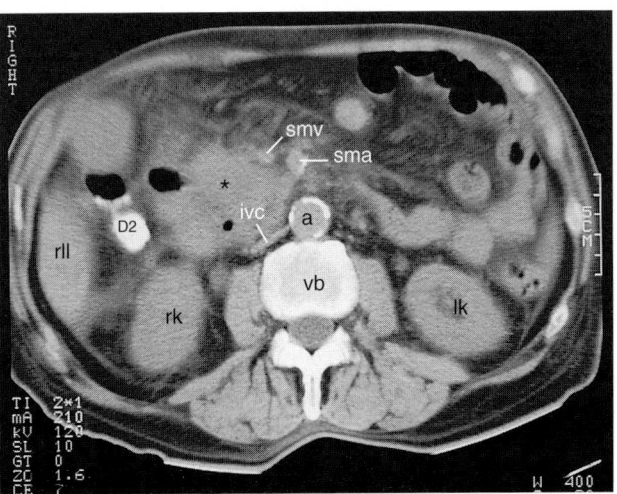

Fig. 4.30 CT pancreas, carcinoma of pancreatic head (*). rk: right kidney, lk: left kidney, vb: vertebral body, a: aorta, ivc: inferior vena cava, D2: second part of duodenum, smv: superior mesenteric vein, sma: superior mesenteric artery.

- Local node enlargement.*
- Local organ invasion.*
- Metastases.*

(*These indicate non-resectability)

Because of the non-specific appearances of a focal pancreatic lesion, percutaneous fine needle aspiration cytology or core biopsy is often required to confirm the diagnosis.

FOCAL LIVER LESIONS

The other strength of ultrasound in biliary scanning is that discrete masses can be identified within the liver. Some are said to have a typical appearance (e.g. a 'target lesion' associated with metastatic deposition) but, generally speaking, the information obtained is:

1. The size of the lesion
2. The internal structure of the lesion
   simple cyst
   complex cyst (i.e. internal bands or debris)
   solid.

Metastases

The diagnosis is usually straightforward with multiple lesions and an appropriate clinical presentation (although it may be more challenging, with a single lesion). On ultrasound the lesion is hypoechoic, and may have a 'target' appearance (**Fig. 4.31a**). On CT the attenuation is lower than that of the surrounding liver parenchyma (**Fig. 4.31b**), and on MRI metastases are of decreased signal on T1W and increased signal on T2W pulse sequences. As a rule of thumb, on MRI of

the liver, metastases are of the same signal as the spleen, regardless of the sequence (**Fig. 4.31c**).

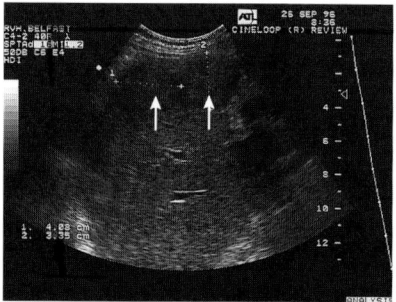

Fig. 4.31(a) Liver metastasis (target lesion), ultrasound.

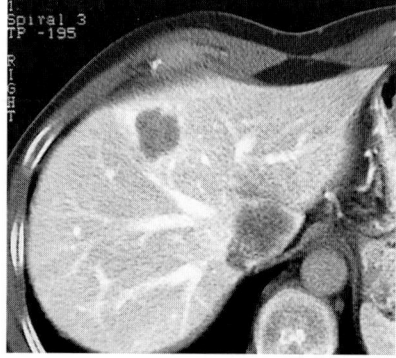

Fig. 4.31(b) Liver metastases, CT.

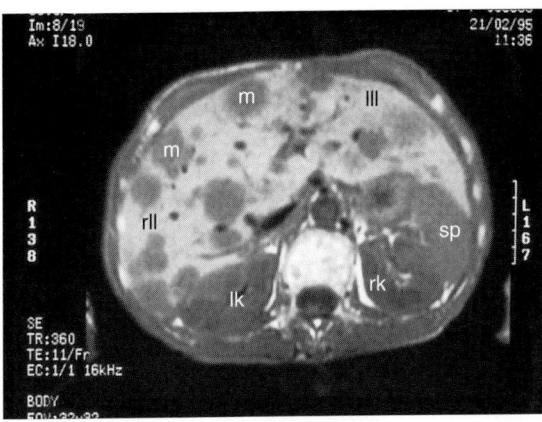

Fig. 4.31(c) MRI: Liver Metastases. m: metastases, sp: spleen, rk: right kidney, lk: left kidney, lll: left lobe liver, rll: right lobe liver.

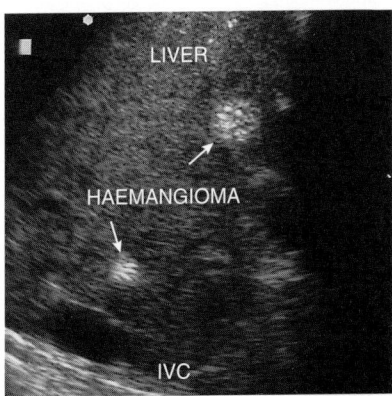

Fig. 4.32 Haemangioma of liver: ultrasound.

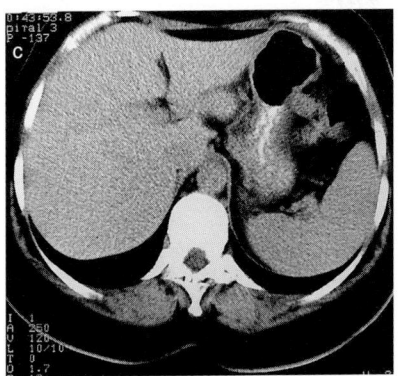

Fig. 4.33(a)

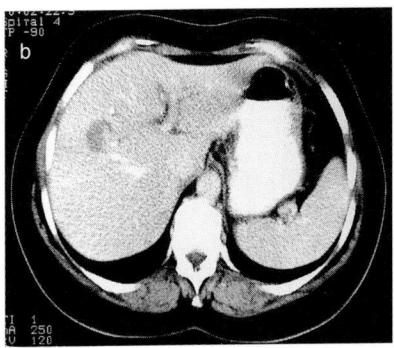

Fig. 4.33 Haemangioma: CT appearances. **a**, The haemangioma (h) initially appears as a low attennative lesion. After a few minutes, **b**, there is wall enhancement, and 20 minutes later, **c**, the lesion has become isointense with the liver, i.e. 'disappeared'.

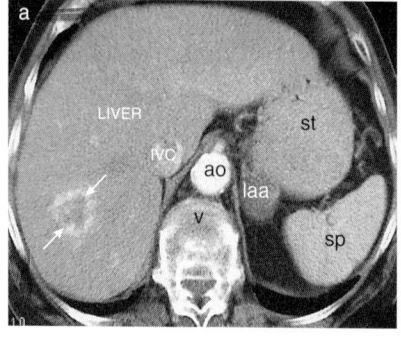
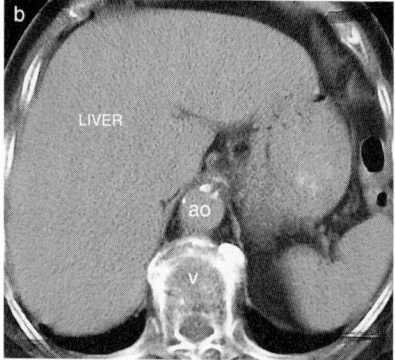

Fig. 4.34 Haemangioma, bright lobe of liver: delayed CT appearances. (a) The initial scan is enhanced. Note the enhancement of the edge of the haemangioma. The brightness is the same as the aorta. (b) 10 minutes later the lesion has vanished.

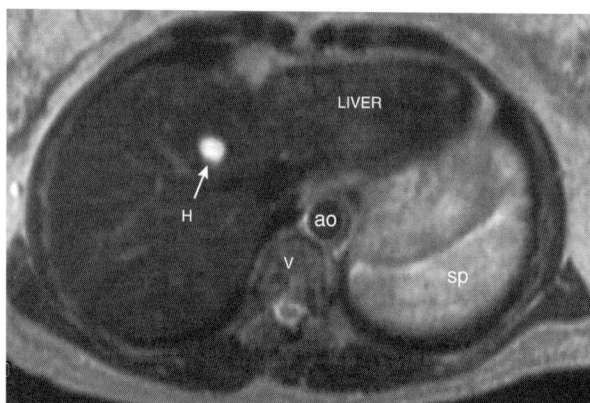

Fig. 4.35
Haemangioma: MRI appearance.

Haemangiomas

Haemangiomata are seen as hyper-echoic (bright), well-defined circular lesions within the liver parenchyma on ultrasound. They have a distinctive appearance on ultrasound (**Fig. 4.32;** p. 63), but on unenhanced CT they may be indistinguishable from a metastatic deposit. Fortunately, however, haemangiomata can usually be differentiated from liver metastases by their physical characteristics on contrast enhanced CT or MRI. On delayed enhanced CT image sequences (**Fig. 4.33a, b, c** [p. 63] **and 4.34a, b**), the haemangioma 'disappears'. On MRI the haemangioma exhibits a very high signal against the low signal background of the liver (**Fig. 4.35**). Less than 2% of metastases have these characteristics.

Further Reading

Adam A, Gibson R N 1994 Interventional radiology of the hepatobiliary and gastrointestinal tract. London: Edward Arnold.

Webb W R, Brant W E, Helms C A 1991 Fundamentals of body CT. Philadelphia: W B Saunders.

5 | Urological Radiology

In this chapter, emphasis is laid on the appearances of the renal tracts in the intravenous urogram (IVU). However, as access to sonography becomes more prevalent, consideration is given to ultrasonic and Doppler appearances.

EVALUATION OF THE NORMAL IVU

Normal anatomy

The adult kidneys measure 11–15 cm in longitudinal diameter on plain radiographs. This equates to 3.5 vertebral bodies plus the intervening discs. On ultrasound, the kidneys appear a little smaller (10–12 cm in longitudinal diameter) (**Fig. 5.1**). This is because the IVU and plain radiographs magnify the image by 20%. The bladder is anechoic on ultrasound (**Fig. 5.2**).

The left kidney may be larger than the right by 0.5 cm. A difference in size of more than 1.5 cm is abnormal. The parenchymal thickness is 2 cm at the midportion and up to 3.5 cm at the poles (**Figs 5.3–5.5**; p. 67–68). The right kidney tends to be lower than the left because of the bulk of the liver, but in 10% of patients the right kidney is higher.

NORMAL VARIANTS

The kidney develops in the pelvis and migrates cranially. Its initial blood supply is from the iliac artery, and it has a further transitional supply before being finally vascularized by the renal artery. The glomeruli and the proximal duct system develop

65

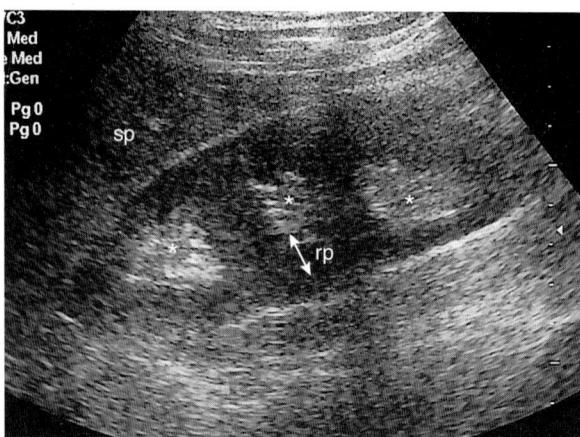

Fig. 5.1 Ultrasound of kidney: longitudinal view of the left kidney. sp: spleen, rp: renal parenchyma, *: renal sinus echoes (collecting system).

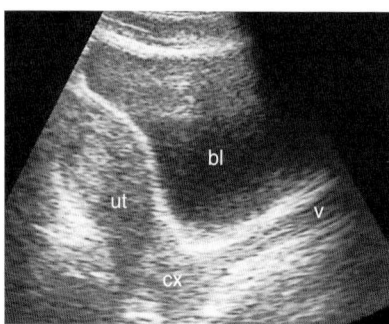

Fig. 5.2 Ultrasound of bladder (bl): sagittal section, female pelvis. ut: uterus, cx: cervix, v: vagina.

from the metanephros, and the collecting tubules, calyces, renal pelvis and the ureter from the metanephric duct.

The kidney
Congenital absence of a kidney
This occurs in 1 : 1000 live births.

Duplex kidneys
Duplication of the renal pelvis occurs in 10% of the population. It can be associated with ureteric duplication, either partial or complete. This is caused by duplication of the metanephric bud by the mesonephric duct (**Figs 5.6–5.8**).

Duplex kidneys

- Distribution equal: right = left
- Male : female ratio 2 : 1
- Bilateral in 20%.

The Weigart-Meyer law

There is an inverse relationship between ureteric insertion and the position of the renal segments of each ureter. The ureter draining the upper pole of the kidney opens medially and inferior to the ureter draining the lower renal pole. It is the upper moiety that obstructs, and the lower moiety that refluxes (the *drooping flower*, **Fig. 5.9**; p. 70).

An ectopic ureterocoele is seen in 70% of duplex kidneys.

Renal ectopia

In utero, as the kidney migrates cranially to its final location on the posterior abdominal wall, it can stop along the embryonic pathway (**Fig. 5.10a, b**; p. 70). The kidney can also continue upward ascent to become a thoracic kidney. This usually occurs through a congenital (through a left posterior or Bochdalek hernia) defect in the diaphragm.

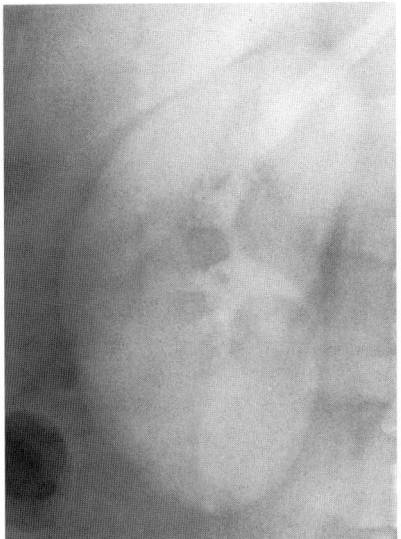
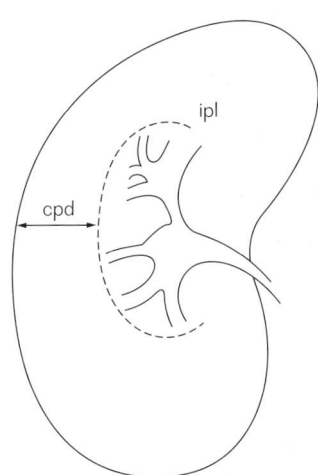

Fig. 5.3 IVU: nephrogram. Typically a few minutes after the injection of i.v. contrast, the renal outline is apparent. In this image the calyceal system has opacified, allowing the interpapillary line (ipl) to be identified and corticopapillary distance (cpd) measured.

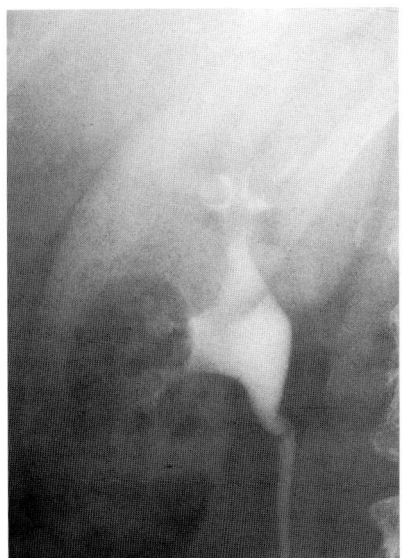
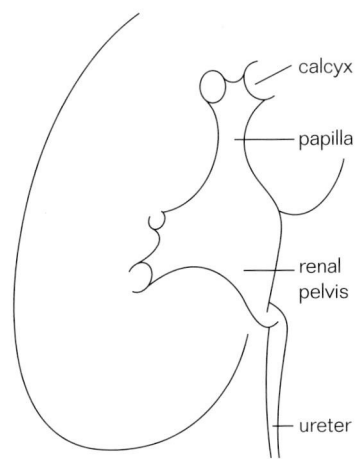

Fig. 5.4 IVU: the pelvicalyceal system. A few minutes after the nephrogram stage, filling of the renal pelvis and ureter is seen distinctly. The calyces are normally said to be 'cupped' and this is produced by indentation of the pyramid. Diseases of the calyces cause 'clubbing'.

Crossed ectopia

Crossed ectopia occurs when the kidney migrates to the opposite side of the abdomen while the vesicoureteric junction remains on the ipsilateral side. In 90% of cases the crossing kidney fuses to the

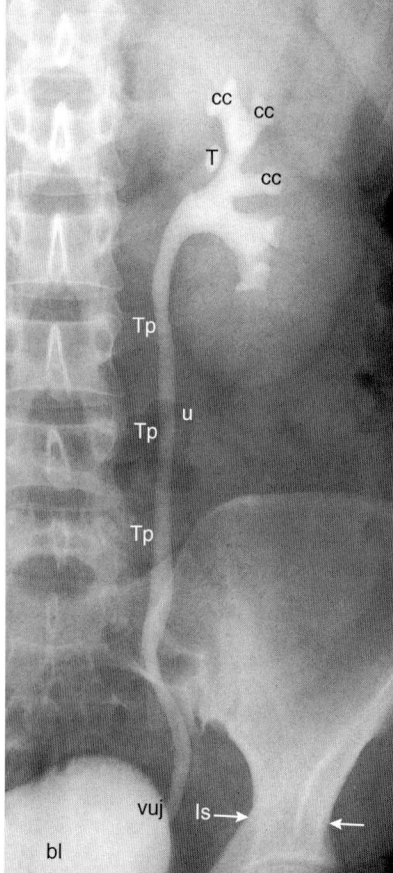

Fig. 5.5 Full-length IVU. The ureters classically run along the transverse processes (Tp) of the vertebral bodies. In this patient the left ureter (u) is obstructed at the vesicoureteric junction (vuj). Consequently the calyces are enlarged and less sharply defined (clubbed) (cc). Note the prominent density produced by a tablet (T) in the patient's stomach. IS: level of ischial spine, bl: bladder.

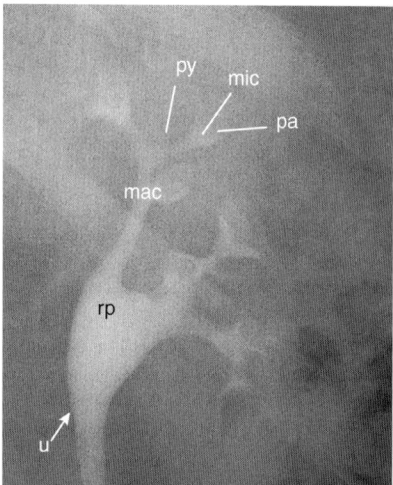

Fig. 5.6 IVU showing normal renal pelvis, compare with **5.7a** (duplex kidney). py: pyramid, mic: minor calyx, mac: major calyx, pa: papilla, rp: renal pelvis, u: ureter.

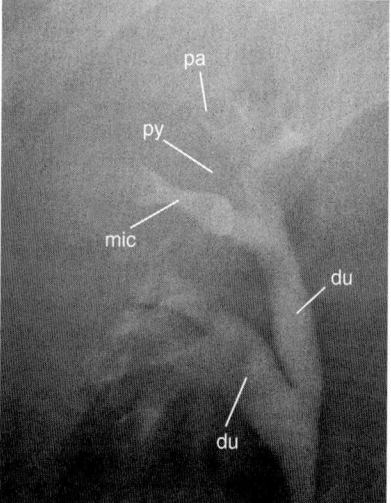

Fig. 5.7(a) IVU showing duplex renal pelvis. py: pyramid, mic: minor calyx, pa: papilla, du: duplication.

lower pole of the opposite kidney, and this is termed *crossed fused ectopia* (**Fig. 5.11a, b; p. 71**).

Fusion abnormalities

The most common fusion abnormality is the *horseshoe kidney* with an incidence of between 1 : 400 and 1 : 750. In this abnormality parenchyma, or fibrous tissue, fuses the lower poles of the two kidneys. This is caused by fusion of the metanephric masses during development. The kidneys are low, with the renal pelvis pointing

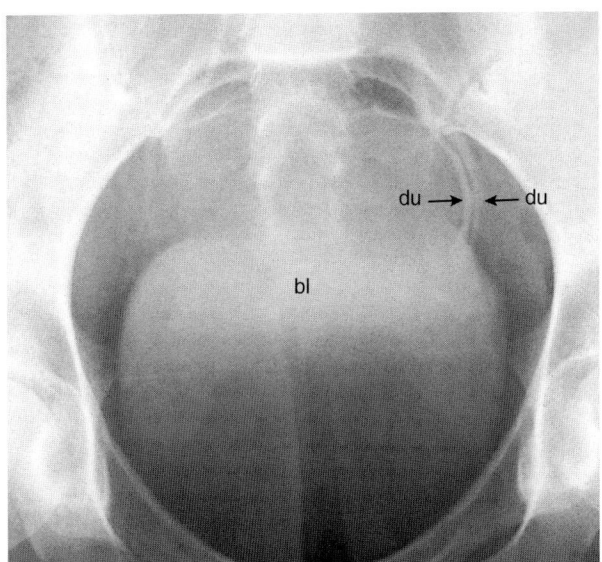

Fig. 5.7(b) IVU showing duplex ureters.
du: duplex ureter,
bl: bladder.

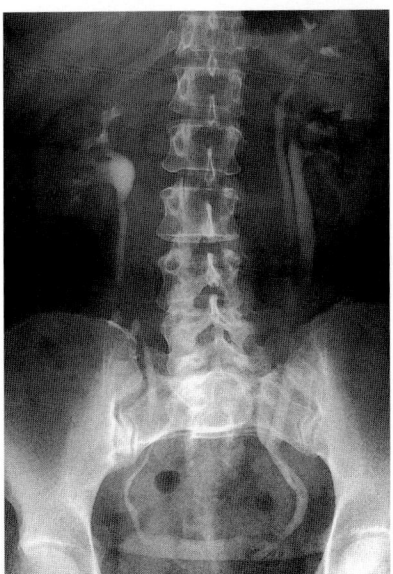

Fig. 5.8 Duplex kidney and ureter. There is a single ureter on the right and complete ureteric duplication on the left. Note that the duplex left kidney is larger than the right kidney.

anteriorly, and the calyces medially. Of note, the vascular supply is anomalous, with vessels supplying the parenchyma from multiple aortic or iliac sites (**Figs 5.12–5.14;** p. 72–73).

The ureter

The ureter is 25–30 cm long, 3 mm wide and develops as a blind diverticulum from the metanephric duct. The intravesical portion of the ureter has an oblique 2 cm course through the bladder wall. Duplication occurs in 2–4% of the population.

Vascular impression

This may cause mild dilatation of the ureter proximal to the impression.

Sites of vascular impression

- Proximal ureter
  Normal/abnormal renal arteries (Fraley's syndrome; **Fig. 5.15;** p. 73)
- Middle ureter
  Iliac vessels at L5/S1. Occasionally the ureter is retroiliac.

Retrocaval ureter

This occurs as a result of persistence of the right subcardinal vein in the development

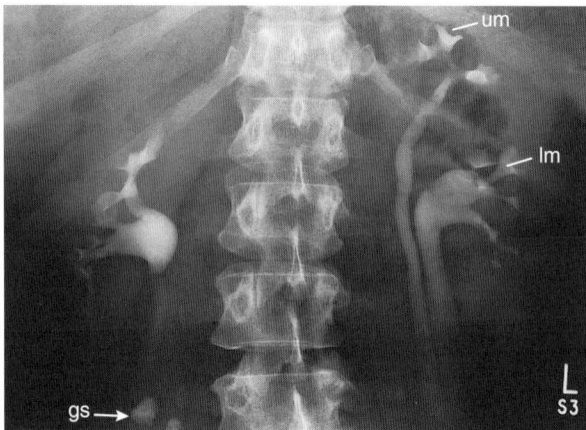

Fig. 5.9 Duplex kidney: the drooping flower. lm: lower moiety (aka the dropping flower), um: upper moiety.

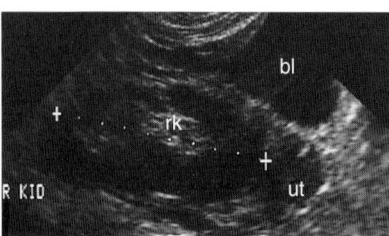

Fig. 5.10(a) Pelvic kidney: ultrasound. rk: right kidney, ut: uterus, bl: bladder.

of the inferior vena cava (IVC). The retrocaval ureter usually occurs at L3, and on the IVU appears as a 'hook-like' medial displacement of the ureter (**Fig. 5.16**; p. 74). This is also known as the low-loop, or type 1 (90%). There is also a high-loop type, or type 2, at the same level as the renal pelvis.

The retrocaval ureter is located posteriorly and medially to the IVC. On the left (although much more rarely) a retroaortic ureter can occur.

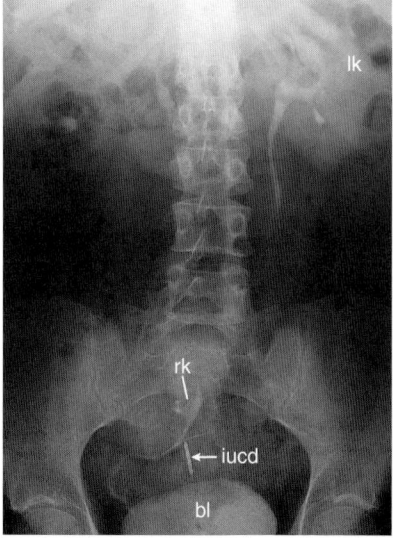

Fig. 5.10(b) Pelvic kidney: IVU. Note the intrauterine contraceptive device (iucd). rk: right kidney, ut: uterus, bl: bladder, lk: left kidney.

RENAL CALCULI

Renal calculi are of varying visibility, ranging from opaque calcium-containing to non-opaque calculi. They are therefore of variable detection on plain radiograph (**Fig. 5.17**; p. 74).

1. Opaque calculi
   (a) Calcium oxalate
   (b) Calcium ammonium magnesium phosphate (struvite): calcium oxalate stones are more radiopaque

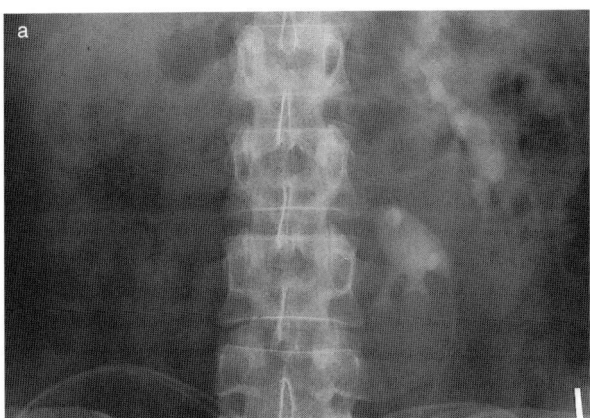

Fig. 5.11 a Crossed fused ectopia: IVU.

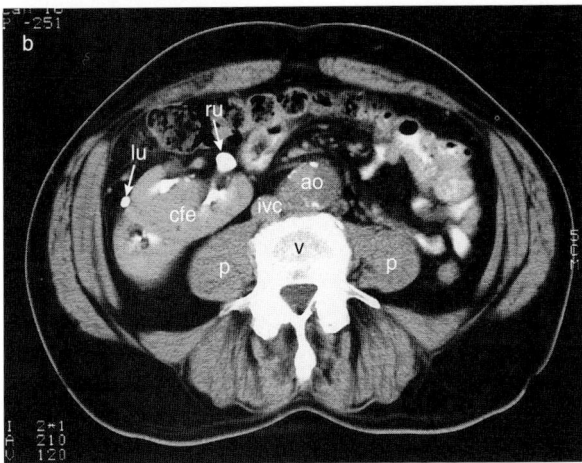

Fig. 5.11 b Crossed fused ectopia: CT. Note the small aortic aneurysm (ao). ru: right ureter, lu: left ureter, cfe: crossed fused ectopic kidney, ivc: inferior vena cava, p: psoas muscle, v: vertebral body.

than triple phosphate (struvite) stones. These struvite stones occur more commonly with alkaline urine. Calcium-containing stones may occur secondary to any cause of hypercalcaemia. If the serum calcium is normal, this suggests intrinsic renal pathology, secondary to either an anatomical or a pathological process (**Fig. 5.18**; p. 74).

2. Poorly opaque stones: cysteine stones. These occur in cystinuria.

3. Non-opaque stones: xanthine, uric acid and matrix stones.

Renal stones and inflammatory bowel disease

Oxalate stones are associated with Crohn's disease because normally, in the small bowel, oxalate binds to calcium making it insoluble and therefore not suitable for reabsorption. In malabsorption, calcium binds to fat and therefore soluble oxalate remains and can be reabsorbed in the colon. (CrOhns = Oxalate stones.)

Uric acid stones can occur as a result of a large volume of diarrhoea and effluent at an iliostomy, which predisposes to acid urine. This urine becomes concentrated,

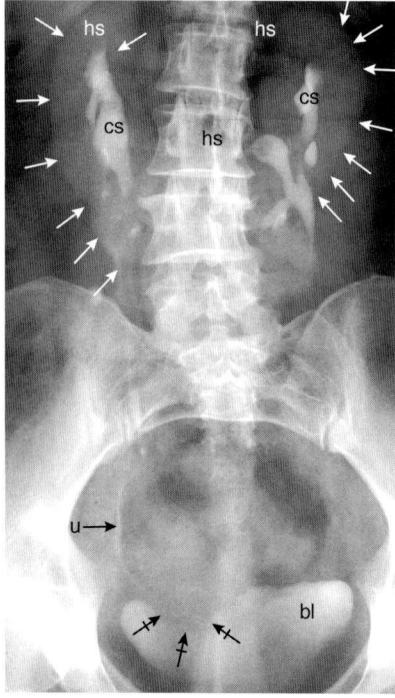

Fig. 5.12 Horseshoe kidney (hs): IVU. cs: collecting system, u: ureter, bl: bladder, arrows: outline of horseshoe kidney. Note the normal smooth impression made by anteverted uterus on the bladder (crossed arrows).

urate becomes crystallized and stones form. (**U**lcerative colitis = **U**rate stones.)

Xanthine stones tend to form due to a failure of the normal oxidation of purines, as in xanthine oxidase deficiency.

Ischial spine rule

Densities identified below a line drawn between the ischial spines are generally too low to be in the ureter. Other causes of such densities would include phleboliths and calcified lymph nodes (**Figs 5.19 and 5.20**; p. 75).

Suggested algorithm for the investigation of renal calculi

Renal calculi associated with colic

The IVU is indicated while the pain is present. Some centres use the combination of ultrasound and a plain film in renal colic. Ultrasound will demonstrate the hydronephrosis and is also useful for those at increased risk from irradiation or intravenous contrast media. Plain films alone are of minimal value.

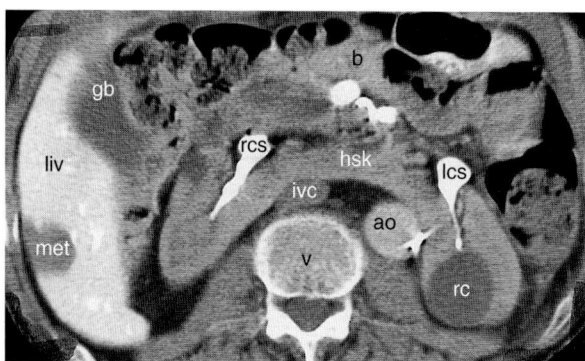

Fig. 5.13 Horseshoe kidney: CT. Note the renal cyst (rc) on the left side of the horseshoe kidney (hsk) and the metastasis (met) on the right lobe of the liver. (The examination was performed to stage colorectal cancer; the horseshoe kidney was an incidental finding.) b: bowel, gb: gallbladder, liv: liver, rcs: right collecting system, lcs: left collecting system, ivc: inferior vena cava, ao: aorta (containing a pigtail catheter), v: vertebral body.

Renal calculi in the absence of pain

The plain abdominal radiograph may be adequate to track calculi following the acute attack. Again, ultrasound will confirm the presence of hydronephrosis.

HAEMATURIA

Haematuria may be macroscopic or microscopic. The commonest causes are listed in **Table 5.1** (p. 75). Regardless of the type of haematuria, one of the most important considerations for the clinican is the age of the patient. *Note:* The degree of haematuria does not correlate with the patho-logical severity; and the incidence of microscopic and macroscopic haematuria is not affected by therapeutic anticoagulation. Do not assume this to be the cause.

Imaging methodology

Each of the two commonly used modalities, the IVU and ultrasound, has its own strengths. Ultrasound is more sensitive at detecting small bladder lesions (0.5 mm) than the IVU (see **Fig. 5.27;** p. 79). The IVU is better at detecting ureteric disease (**Fig. 5.21;** p. 76). Furthermore, the risk of serious underlying cause of haematuria increases after 40 years of age. Many authors advocate cystoscopy in this age group anyway; therefore the increased sensitivity of ultrasound is less of an advantage.

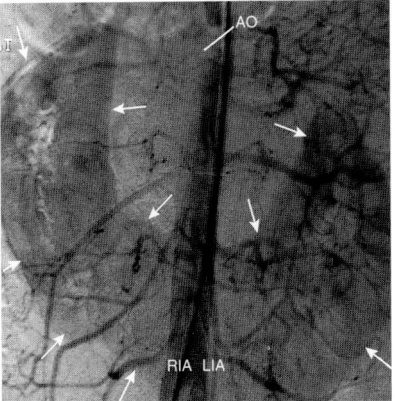

Fig. 5.14 Horseshoe kidney: angiogram. AO: aorta, RIA: right iliac artery, LIA: left iliac artery, arrows: outline of horseshoe kidney.

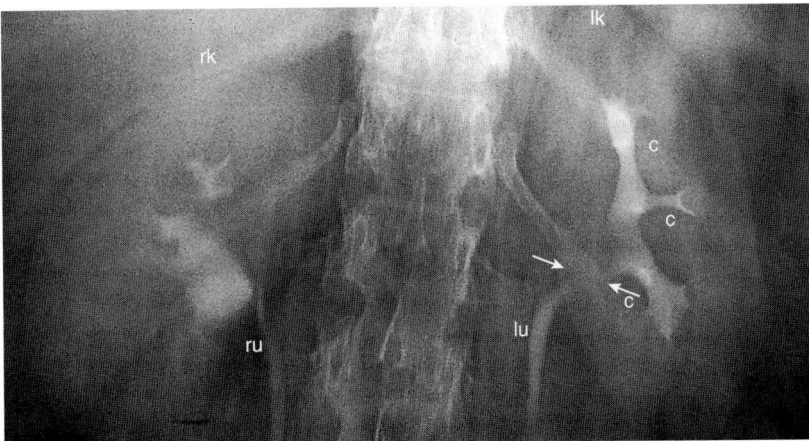

Fig. 5.15 Fraley's syndrome: IVU. Note that there is no dilatation of the left renal collecting system by the vascular impression (arrows). In this patient, the right kidney (rk) outlines normally. lk: left kidney, lu: left ureter, ru: right ureter, c: calyces.

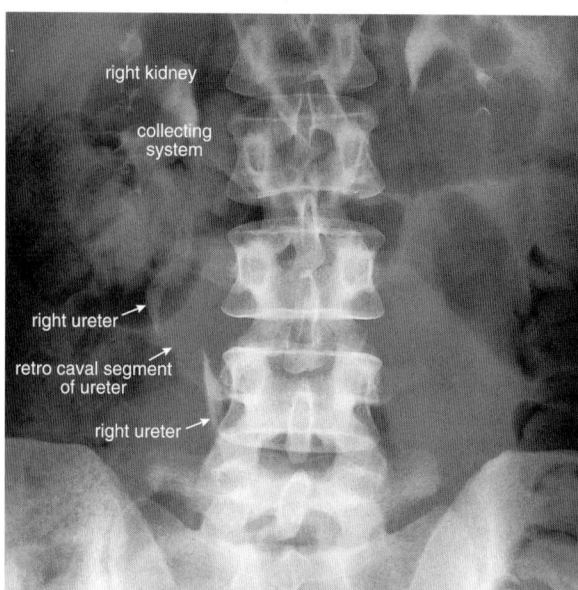

Fig. 5.16 Retrocaval ureter: IVU.

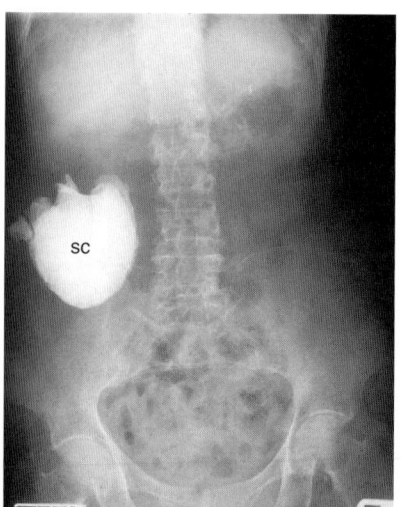

Fig. 5.17 Staghorn calculus (sc): plain abdominal radiograph.

Suggested imaging protocol for haematuria

- Patient <40 years old: ultrasound of renal tracts
- Patient >40 years old: IVU and cystoscopy.

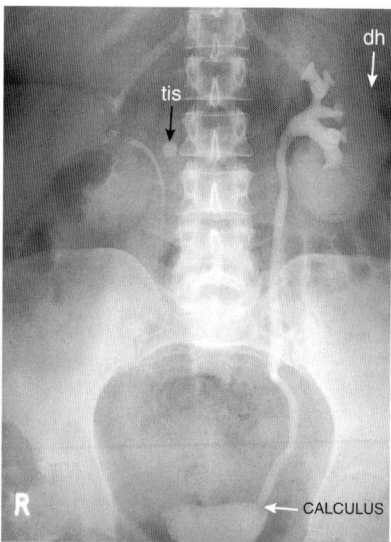

Fig. 5.18 Obstructing calculus within the distal left ureter causing renal colic (IVU). Note the tablet in the stomach (tis) to the right of the L2 vertebral body and the 'dromedary hump' (dh) – a normal convex bump on the lateral aspect of the left kidney. Neither is of significance.

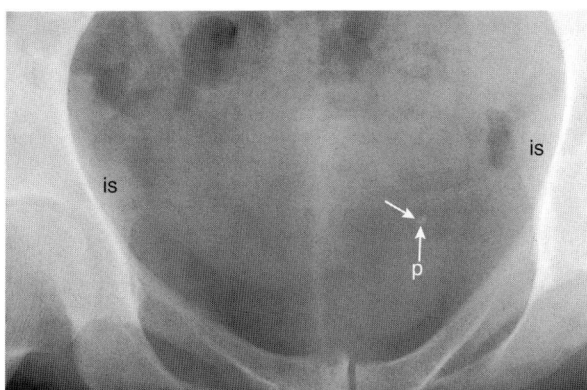

Fig. 5.19 Left-sided phlebolith (p) below the level of the ischial spine (is). it: ischial tuberosity.

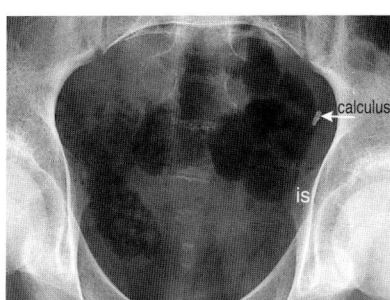

Fig. 5.20 Right-sided ureteric calculus above the level of the ischial spine.

Table 5.1	Aetiology of haematuria		
Microscopic haematuria	**Incidence (%)**	**Macroscopic haematuria**	**Incidence (%)**
Renal cancer	0.5	Renal cancer	4
Ureteric cancer	0.2	Ureteric cancer	1
Bladder cancer	4	Bladder cancer	15
Prostate cancer	0.5	Prostate cancer	2
Urinary tract infection	5	Urinary tract infection	10
Prostatic hypertrophy	13	Prostatic hypertrophy	15
No cause	40	No cause	10

Sutton JM. Evaluation of haematuria in adults. JAMA 1990; 263: 2475–2480.

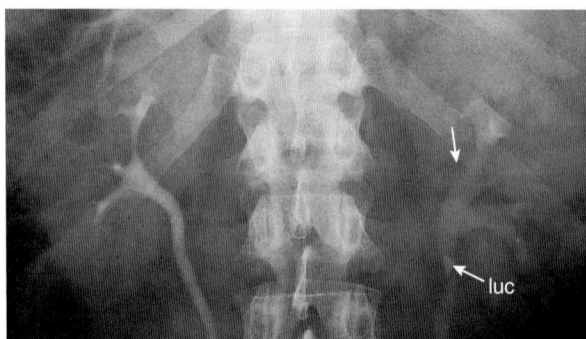

Fig. 5.21 Left hydronephrosis due to ureteric calculus: IVU. luc: left uteric calculus.

TUMOURS OF THE URINARY TRACT

Kidney

The renal cell carcinoma (hypernephroma, renal adenocarcinoma) accounts for 80–90% of all renal malignancies. Five percent are bilateral. On plain radiograph, calcification (in 10%), distortion of the normal renal outline and evidence of secondary bony metastases may be seen.

On ultrasound, the tumour is usually of a different echo texture (it may be brighter or darker) than the normal renal parenchyma (**Fig. 5.22**). CT (pre-contrast) demonstrates a heterogeneous mass with low attenuation areas (representing haemorrhage and necrosis) and dystrophic calcification. Although the tumour is vascular, the enhancement still tends to be less than that of the normal renal tissue. Perinephric invasion, nodes and venous invasion (renal vein, 30%, IVC 5–10%) can be identified (**Fig. 5.23**).

Ureter

Less than 2% of urinary tumours occur in the ureter. Eighty percent of these, however, are malignant, and the transitional cell tumour is the most prevalent. They are usually identified on ultrasound by the accompanying hydronephrosis (**Fig. 5.24**), and

the level can be demonstrated on the IVU (**Fig. 5.25**; p. 78). CT will confirm the level and allow staging of the disease (**Fig. 5.26**; p. 78).

Bladder

The vast majority of tumours are epithelial, transitional cell cancers. Ultrasound will identify more than 90% of tumours greater than 5 mm in size (**Fig. 5.27**; p. 79), and its sensitivity greatly exceeds that of the IVU. On CT, the lesions may be seen as polypoid or sessile projections into the bladder, but may only appear as localized thickenings of the bladder wall. The main indication for CT is for the staging, not detection of the lesion. Both CT and

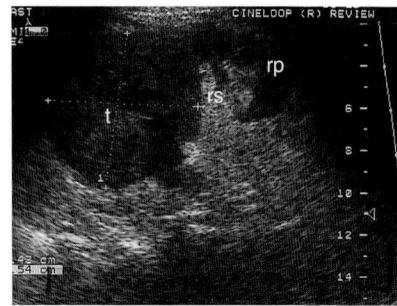

Fig. 5.22 Renal cell carcinoma: ultrasound. rp: renal parenchyme, t: tumour, rs: renal sinus.

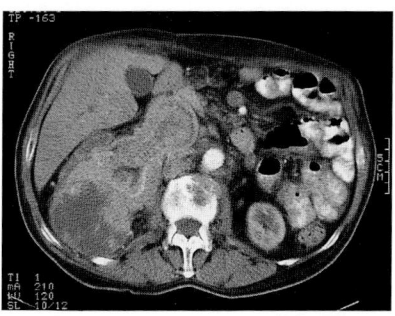 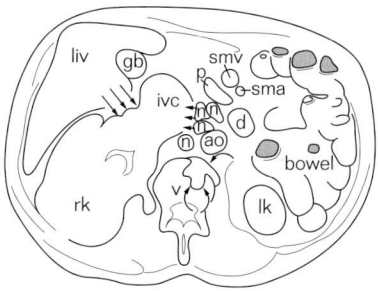

Fig. 5.23 Renal cell carcinoma: CT. There is a large tumour of the right kidney (rk), which has invaded the left renal vein (arrows) and the inferior vena cava (ivc). Both are massively enlarged. Note also the vertebral metastatic deposit (curved arrows) infiltrating the left side of the vertebral body (v). Multiple lymph nodes (n) are noted between the aorta (ao) and the IVC. liv: liver, gb: gallbladder, p: pancreas, d: fourth part of duodenum, smv: superior mesenteric vein, sma: superior mesenteric artery, lk: left kidney.

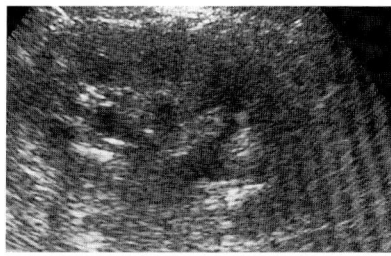 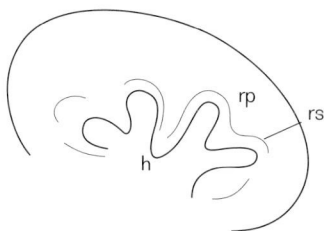

Fig. 5.24 Hydronephrosis: ultrasound. The black central area (h) represents accumulated urine in the hydronephrotic kidney. The renal parenchyma (rp) is darker than the fat in the renal sinus (rs). Persistent 'darkness' within the renal sinus fat should raise the possibility of fluid accumulation.

MRI have an accuracy of 70% in the extravesical staging of bladder malignancy.

Testis

Ultrasound is the imaging modality of choice in the evaluation of scrotal pathol-ogy. The vast majority of testicular mass lesions (90%) are malignant. They appear as hypoechoic (dark) solid areas within the testis (**Fig. 5.28**; p. 79).

URETHRAL INJURIES

The anatomy of the urethra is complex, and a schematic diagram is given in **Figure 5.29** (p. 80).

The anterior urethra (penile and bulbous)

Anterior injuries are infrequent. The anterior urethra is not usually damaged by a

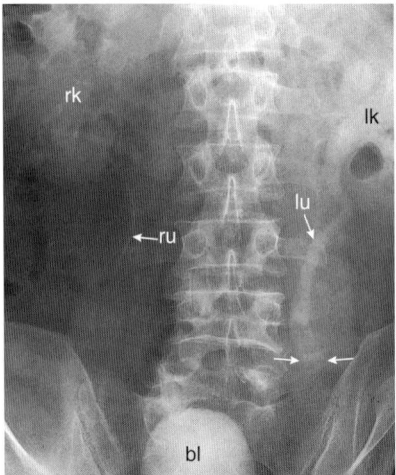

Fig. 5.25 IVU: left ureteric obstruction by tumour. Note the diameter of the hydronephrotic left ureter (lu) compared to the right (ru). The level of the obstruction is marked by arrows. rk: right kidney, lk: left kidney, bl: bladder.

pelvic fracture. Injuries are usually due to direct injury to the penis. The bulbous urethra is crushed against the pelvic floor.

Classification of anterior urethral injuries (i.e. those below the urogenital diaphragm)

- Contusions: no mucosal tears
- Partial: some mucosa bridging the gap
- Complete: transection of the urethra, no continuity of the mucosa

Diagnosis: retrograde urethrogram.

A normal urethrogram rules out an anterior urethral injury, but not a bladder injury. After a normal urethrogram, the catheter may be passed to evaluate the bladder by cystography.

The posterior urethra

Injuries to the posterior urethra are much more common than injuries to the anterior

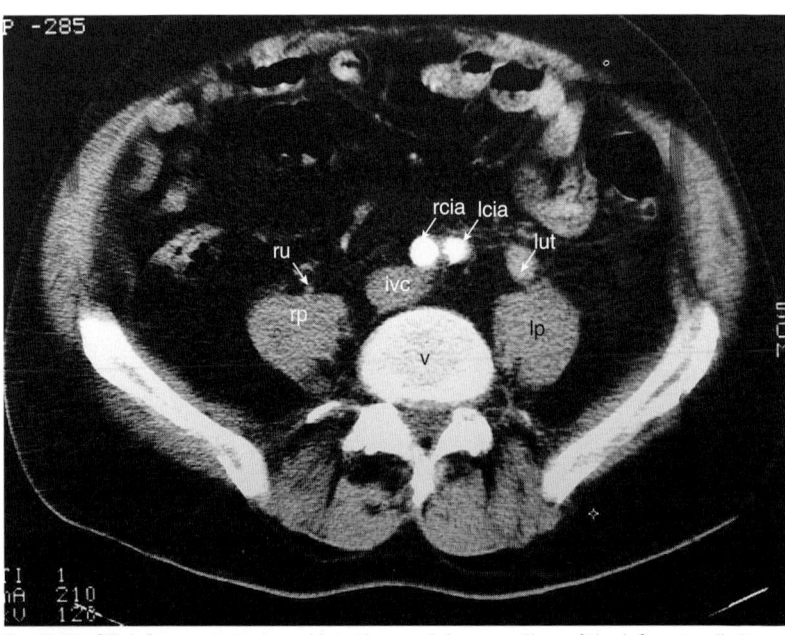

Fig. 5.26 CT: left ureteric tumour. Note the much larger calibre of the left ureter (lut) compared to the right (ru). rcia: right common iliac artery, lcia: left common iliac artery, ivc: inferior vena cava, v: vertebral body, rp: right psoas, lp: left psoas.

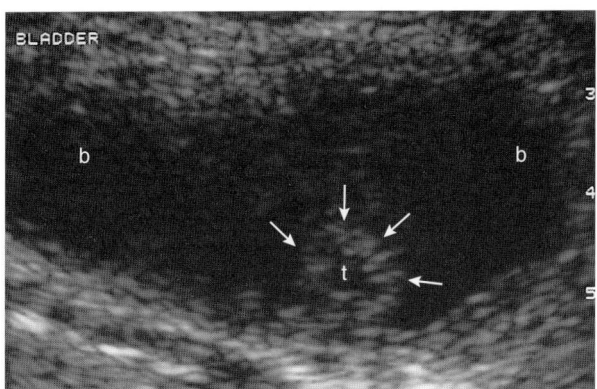

Fig. 5.27 Bladder tumour: ultrasound. This longitudinal image demonstrates a polypoid tumour (t) within the echo-free bladder lumen (b).

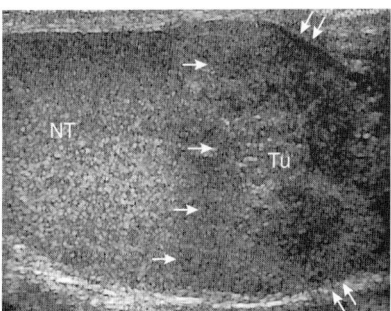

Fig. 5.28 Testicular mass lesion: ultrasound. NT: normal testis, Tu: tumour mass at lower pole of testis.

urethra, and 90% are associated with pelvic fractures. Any male with a pelvic arch fracture should be suspected of having a posterior urethral injury/bladder injury. Such injuries are usually caused by shear force. The membranous urethra is firmly attached to the urogenital diaphragm, but the prostatic urethra is far more mobile owing to its attachment with the mobile pelvic side walls and bladder base.

Therefore, the rapid deceleration results in the posterior urethra being driven back, while the membranous urethra remains firm. The prostatic urethra is shorn at its junction with membranous urethra.

Classification of posterior urethral tears (Colapinto and McCallum)

- Type 1: the posterior urethra is stretched, secondary to haematoma in the prostatic bed. Urethra is intact.
- Type 2: the prostate and urethra are disrupted. The prostatomembranous junction lies above the intact urogenital diaphragm. Extravasation is supradiaphragmatic within the bony pelvis.
- Type 3: both the membranous urethra and the urogenital diaphragm are disrupted, allowing extension of haemorrhage and extravasation from extraperitoneal region of the pelvis into the proximal bulbous urethra.

NON-MALIGNANT SCROTAL PATHOLOGY

Scrotal masses

Ultrasound is the imaging method of choice for the detection of scrotal pathology. Two common scrotal mass lesions include hydroceles and epididymal cysts.

Hydrocele

A hydrocele appears as a black (sonolucent) zone around the testis (**Fig. 5.30**). When it has been present for some time, it typically becomes septated.

79

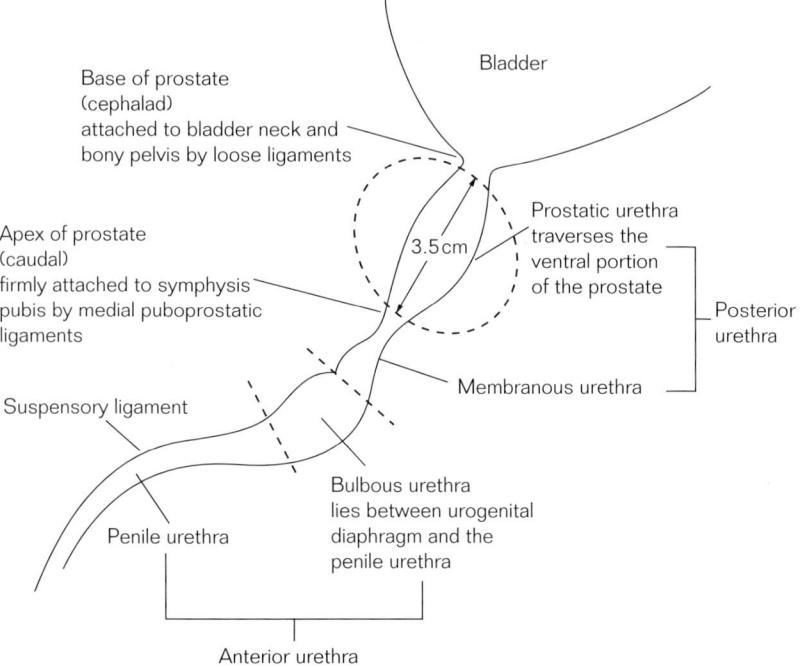

Base of prostate
(cephalad)
attached to bladder neck and
bony pelvis by loose ligaments

Bladder

3.5cm

Prostatic urethra
traverses the
ventral portion
of the prostate

Posterior
urethra

Apex of prostate
(caudal)
firmly attached to symphysis
pubis by medial puboprostatic
ligaments

Membranous urethra

Suspensory ligament

Bulbous urethra
lies between urogenital
diaphragm and the
penile urethra

Penile urethra

Anterior urethra

Fig. 5.29 Anatomy of the urethra.

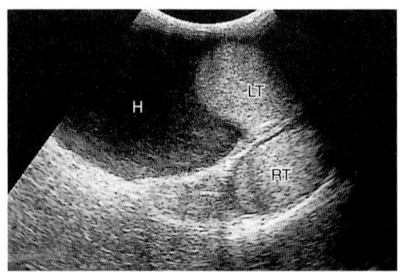

Fig. 5.30 Simple hydrocele (H): ultrasound. LT: left testis, RT: right testis.

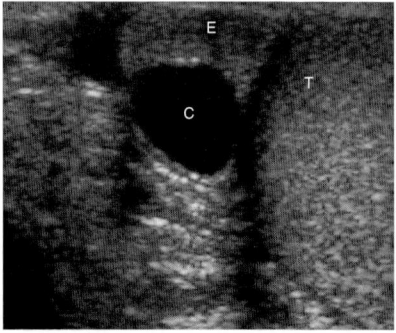

Fig. 5.31 Epididymal cyst (C): ultrasound. T: testis, E: epididymal head.

Epididymal cyst

Cysts of the epididymis are very common. They appear as a circular sonolucent (dark) area, usually within the head of the epididymis (**Fig. 5.31**).

Torsion

Doppler sonography has proved sensitive in identifying flow within intratesticular vessels. However, to date, the consensus is that sonography and Doppler analysis should not be the criterion on which the diagnosis of torsion is based. The diagnosis of testicular torsion remains foremost a clinical diagnosis.

RENAL TRANSPLANTATION

Patients with renal transplants are susceptible to a range of complications.

Cardiovascular complications

- The rate of atherosclerosis is accelerated in renal transplant
- Diabetes occurs in 15% of former non-diabetics
- Renal artery stenosis occurs in 10% of patients (not usually at the anastomosis)
- Hypertension occurs in 50%. This is multifactorial but appears related to:
    native renal pathology
    renal arterial stenosis
    drug nephrotoxicity (cyclosporin)
    graft rejection
- Avascular necrosis. This usually affects the femoral head (10%).

Allograft complications

These may be surgical or medical.

Surgical complications

Perinephric collections: these occur in up to 50% of patients, typically soon after transplantation surgery

Haematomas: usually occur immediately postoperatively, and are complex collections.

Lymphoceles: Seen in 20% of transplants, lymphoceles are large, septated, and usually adjacent to the lower pole of transplant, where they obstruct the ureter. Aspiration alone is rarely successful

Urinomas: Urinomas result from leaks from the ureteroneocystostomy. Treatment is drainage and nephrostomy. The diagnosis is made by scintigraphy.

Obstruction

Ureteric obstruction occurs in up to 8% of transplants (**Fig. 5.32**). This results in hydronephrosis. The commonest cause of obstruction is stenosis of the transplant ureter at the vesicoureteric junction (VUJ). The diagnosis may be made by sonography or CT. (There is normally, however, a degree of calyceal dilatation in the transplanted kidney.) Balloon dilatation of these strictures is successful in up to 75% of cases.

Renal artery stenosis

The gold-standard imaging modality for the diagnosis of renal artery stenosis (RAS) is angiography. However this is invasive, and the non-ionizing alternative of Doppler sonography is widely used.

Doppler criteria for RAS:

1. In the renal artery:
    high-velocity jet
    distal turbulence
2. In the renal parenchyma:
    the *parvus tardus* phenomenon: the parvus tardus waveform describes an arterial waveform that is both weak and delayed (**Fig. 5.33**).

Renal graft dysfunction

Graft dysfunction is usually the result of

- Acute rejection
- Acute tubular necrosis (occurs earliest)

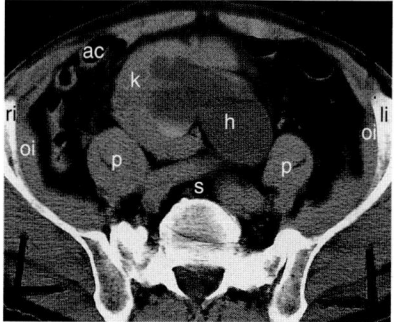

Fig. 5.32 Obstructed transplanted kidney: CT. ri: right innominate bone, li: left innominate bone, s: sacrum, oi: internus muscle, k: kidney, h: hydronephrosis, p: psoas muscle.

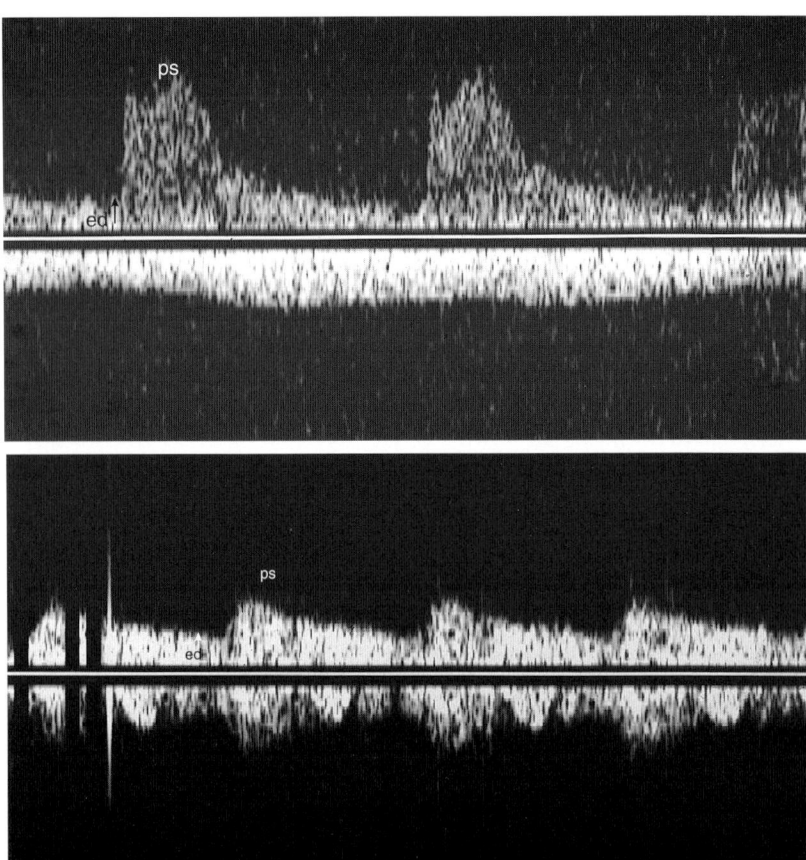

Fig. 5.33 a Normal Doppler arterial renal waveform. Note the steep angle of the wave between and diastolic (ed) and peak systolic (ps) points. **b** the parvus tardus waveform: renal doppler ultrasound. The angle is much less steep (parvus) and the peak comes later (tardus).

- Cyclosporin toxicity.

Biopsy is usually required to differentiate, but there are described features of rejection on ultrasound, which may help with differentiation.

Ultrasound features of rejection

- Kidney enlargement
- Echogenic cortices
- Prominent pyramids

- Hypoechoic renal sinuses
- Decreased diastolic flow in the intrarenal arteries
- Resistive index greater than 0.8 on Doppler.

Renal vein thrombosis

Often secondary to iliac vein thrombosis. High vascular resistance will be demonstrated in the graft, on Doppler ultrasound.

Further Reading

Ell S R 1992 Handbook of gastrointestinal and genitourinary radiology. St Louis: Mosby Year Book.

6 | Radiology of the Spine

> **Topics included in this chapter**
> - Anatomy of the cervical spine
> - Systematic review of the cervical spine radiographs
> - Injuries to the cervical spine
> - Specific cervical spine injuries
> - Thoracolumbar injuries
> - Degenerative diseases
> - Metastases

ANATOMY OF THE CERVICAL SPINE

A vertebra is made up of two components: a vertebral body and a neural arch.

Anterior structures
- Vertebral bodies
- Intervertebral discs
- Longitudinal ligaments
  anterior
  posterior.

The *anterior ligament* is *taut*. It is closely applied to the anterior aspects of the vertebral body and the annulus of the disc. The anterior longitudinal ligament runs from the anterior arch of the atlas to the sacrum and maintains vertebral alignment. The *posterior ligament* is *weaker*. It is applied to the posterior surface of the vertebral bodies and discs.

The neural arch

The neural arch is made up by the posterior elements (pedicle, lamina and transverse process) and the posterior ligament complex. The posterior ligament complex is comprised of the ligamentum flavum, and the interspinous and the supraspinous ligaments. The *ligamentum flavum* lines the dorsal surface of the canal and is *tightly* applied to the laminae. The *interspinous ligaments* interconnect the spinous processes and are overlain by the *supraspinous* ligament.

Biomechanics

The three-column theory of biomechanics divides the cervical spine, as viewed laterally, into three vertical columns: anterior, middle and posterior.

The middle column (posterior longitudinal ligament, posterior part of annulus, and posterior part of vertebral body) acts as the fulcrum connecting the other two. Instability occurs if two of the three columns are damaged.

SYSTEMATIC REVIEW OF THE CERVICAL SPINE RADIOGRAPHS

The lateral cervical spine (**Fig. 6.1**)

Review areas

- Check that the top of the T1 vertebra is seen.
- Trace the five lines. Five lines or arcs can be traced:
  1. Along the prevertebral soft tissues
  2. Along the anterior margins of the vertebral bodies
  3. Along the posterior margins of the vertebral bodies
  4. Along the bases of the spinous processes (spinolaminar line)
  5. Along the tips of the spinous processes.

The prevertebral soft tissues (line 1)

Look for abnormal widening. The posterior wall of nasopharynx should be flat or concave at the level of C2 (**Fig. 6.2**). At the base of the odontoid peg, the thickness of the prevertebral soft tissues should be less than the peg thickness (<4–5 mm) and at the level of the C6 vertebra, the width of a vertebral body (<20 mm). Swelling of the prevertebral tissues occurs in 50% of patients with a cervical bony injury (**Fig. 6.3**).

Anterior and posterior vertebral lines (lines 2 and 3)

As a rule (for both anterior and posterior vertebral lines), more than 3–4 mm of forward movement suggests instability or a unifacet dislocation (see later) and a 40–50% overlap suggests a bifacet dislocation.

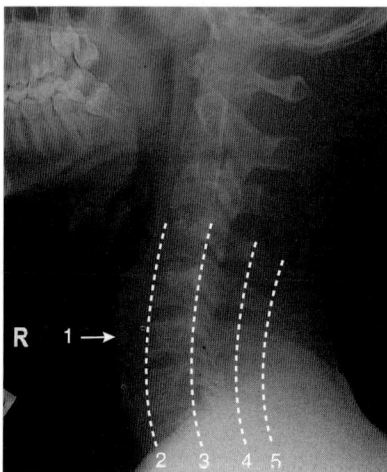

Fig. 6.1 Lateral cervical spine. (1) Prevertebral soft tissues, (2) anterior vertebral line, (3) posterior vertebral line, (4) spinolaminar line, (5) spinous process tips line.

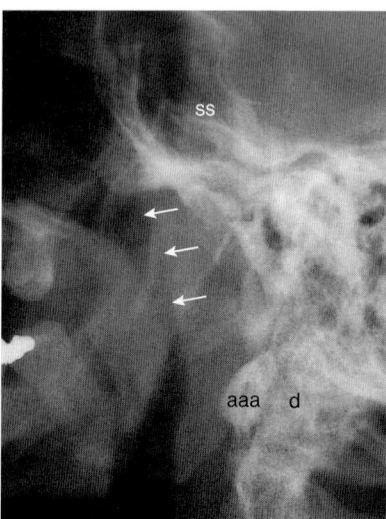

Fig. 6.2 Lateral cervical spine (detail): normal appearance of prevertebral nasopharyngial soft tissue (arrows). Note, however, a fluid level in the sphenoid sinus (ss). This patient had a basal skull fracture. aaa: anterior arch of the atlas, d: dens.

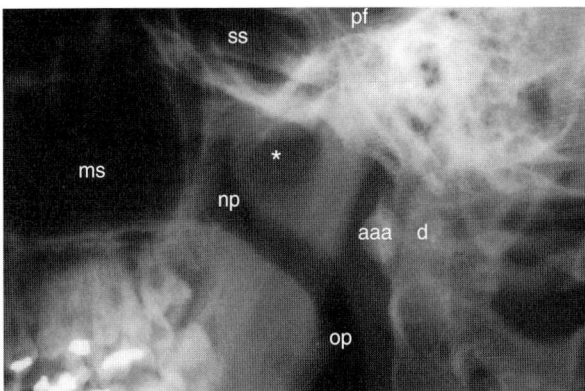

Fig. 6.3 Lateral cervical spine (detail): convex nasopharyngeal shadow. There is abnormal soft tissue in the nasopharynx (*) anterior to the upper cervical vertebrae. aaa: anterior arch of the atlas, d: dens, pf: pituitary fossa, ss: sphenoid sinus, ms: maxillary sinus, np: nasopharynx, op: oropharynx.

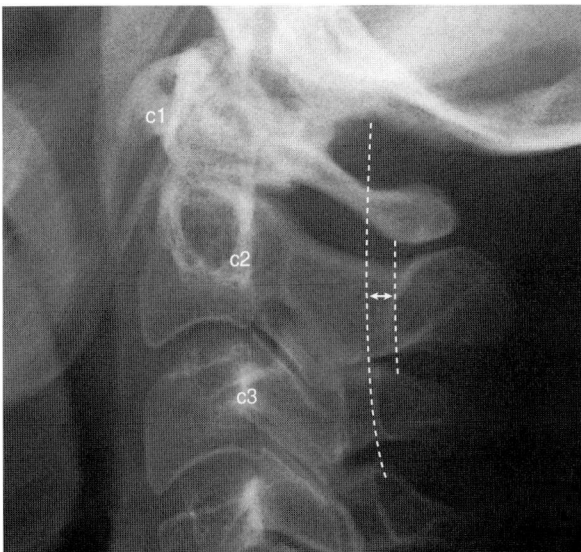

Fig. 6.4 Physiological gap at the spinolaminar line at c2.

Spinolaminar line (line 4)

The spinolaminar line may sometimes show a slight step at C2 particularly in children. This posterior step should not be more than 2 mm behind the smooth arc traced from C3 to C1. More than 2–3 mm disruption at this level suggests disruption of the elastic lamina and the posterior column **(Fig. 6.4)**.

Line through the tips of the spinous processes (line 5)

The distance between the tips of the spinous processes is very variable. However, as a rule, a difference of more than 50% in the distance between the tips should be regarded with caution.

The Power's ratio (**Fig. 6.5**)

Line A joins the tip of the anterior arch of atlas to the posterior lip of the foramen magnum. Line B joins the anterior tip of the foramen magnum to the (spinolaminar) tip of C1. The ratio B:A should be <1. A Power's ratio (B:A) >1 suggests anterior subluxation at the atlanto-occipital junction.

Harris's ring

This is an oval lucency projected through the C2 vertebral body on the lateral view. The superior pole of Harris's ring coincides with the base of the odontoid process. Fractures of the dens cause disruption in the ring (**Fig. 6.6**).

Intervertebral foramina

These are not visible on the lateral view except at C2/3 and C7/T1. If the intervertebral foramen of C6/7 is visible on the lateral view, it suggests thoracization of C7. If seen, suspect a cervical rib (**Figs 6.7–6.9**).

The anterior 'peg' radiograph

The lateral margins of C1 should align with the lateral margins of C2. The space on each side of the odontoid peg should be equal (**Fig. 6.10**). *Exception: slight rotation of the neck may cause these spaces to appear unequal. However, if, in this instance, the lateral margins of C1 and C2 remain normally aligned then this asymmetry may be attributed to rotation.*

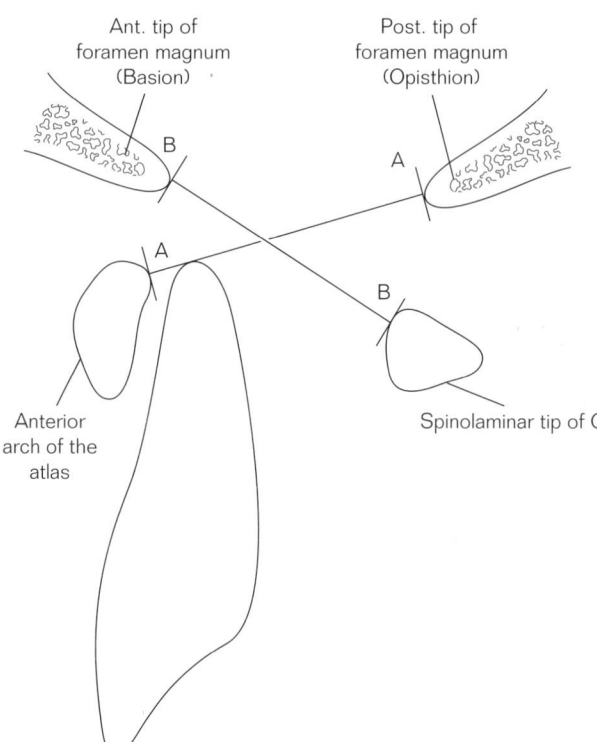

Ant. tip of
foramen magnum
(Basion)

Post. tip of
foramen magnum
(Opisthion)

B

A

A

B

Anterior
arch of the
atlas

Spinolaminar tip of Cl.

Fig. 6.5 Sagittal section through the skull base demonstrating the Power's ratio (normally B/A < 1.

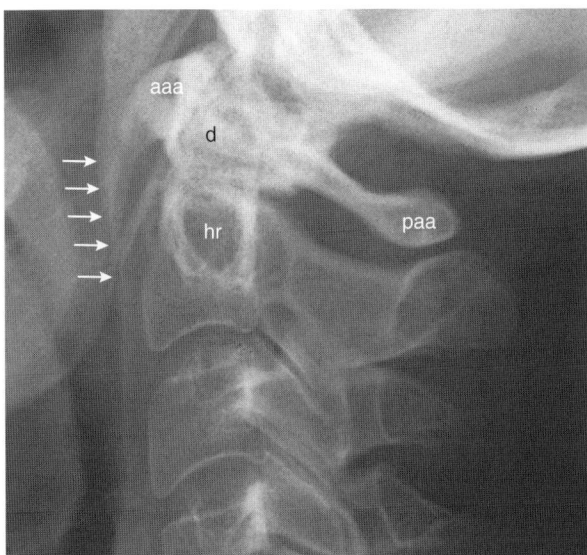

Fig. 6.6 Harris's ring (hr). aaa: anterior arch of atlas, paa: posterior arch of atlas, d: dens, arrows: prevertebral soft tissue.

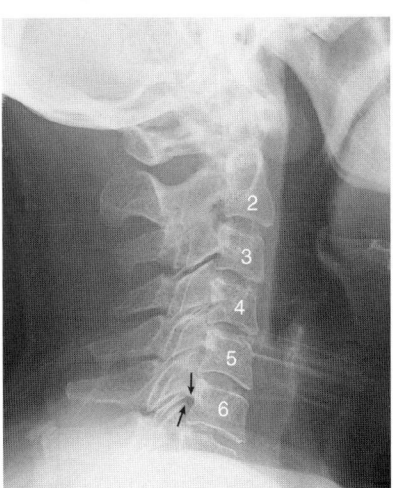

Fig. 6.7 Normal intervertebral foramen at C6/7.

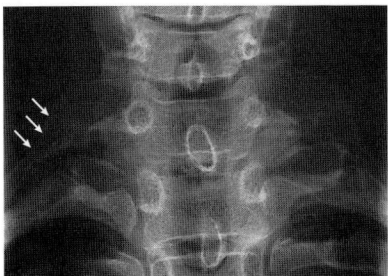

Fig. 6.9 Cervical rib. Anterior cervical spine.

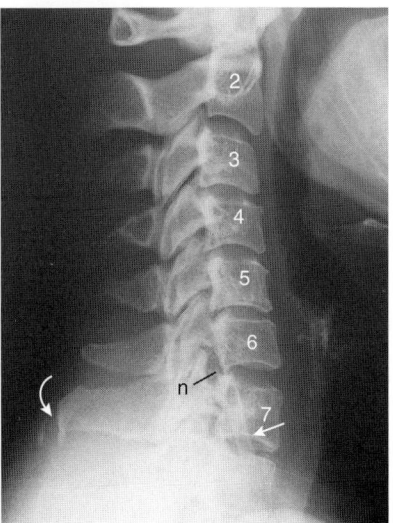

Fig. 6.8 'Thoracic' intervertebral foramen at C6/7 indicating cervical rib. The neurovertebral foramen of C6/7 is prominent (n). This suggests thoracization of the C7 vertebral body. A cervical rib was noted (arrow) and the diagnosis confirmed on the anterior projection. (Note also 'clay shoveller's' fracture of C7 spinous process (curved arrow)).

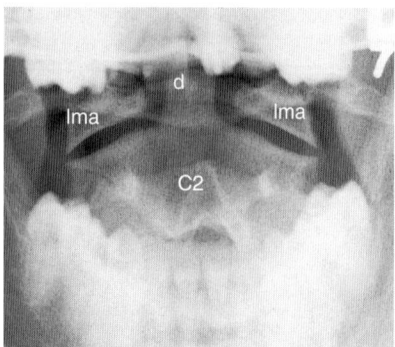

Fig. 6.10 Anterior peg view, cervical spine. Note the normal alignment between the lateral borders of C1 and C2. d: dens, lma: lateral mass of atlas, C2: second vertebral body.

On the open mouth 'peg' view, look for:

- A fracture of the odontoid peg
- The lateral masses of C1 overhanging the lateral margins of C2 (Jefferson fracture)
- Unequal or asymmetric spaces between the odontoid peg and the lateral masses of the atlas.

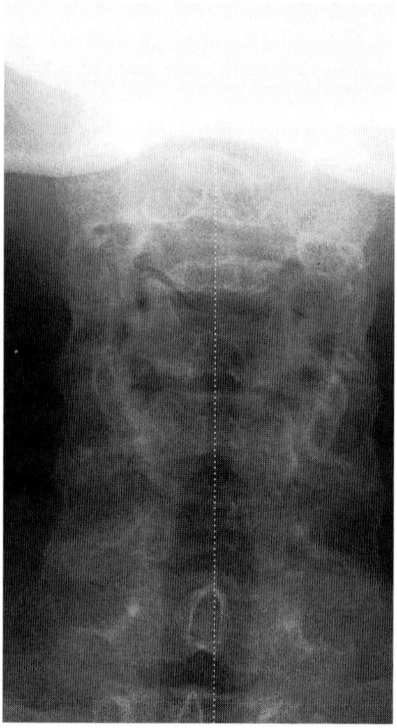

Fig. 6.11 Normal anterior cervical spine radiograph. Note that the spinous processes are all aligned (·····).

The anterior cervical spine (the 'long AP view')

Check the spinous processes: these should be in a straight line (**Fig. 6.11**). Deviation may indicate a unifacetal dislocation. If deviation is detected, scrutinize the lateral view carefully. *Note: the spinous processes may not lie in a straight line when bifid spinous processes are present.* The distance between the spinous processes should be approximately equal. No single space should be more than 50% wider than the one immediately above or below.

INJURIES TO THE CERVICAL SPINE

Injuries are most common in the lower cervical spine (C5–C7, T1) and at the C1/2 articulation. Eight percent of patients have injuries to the cervical canal in more than one place, and 15–20% of patients with a cervical spine fracture have an initially unsuspected second vertebral column fracture. Approximately 20% of spinal fractures are associated with fractures elsewhere in the body. Spinal cord injuries occur in

10–14% of spinal fractures and dislocations. In cervical spine fractures, there is a 40% incidence of associated neurological injury, and in patients sustaining fractures of the vertebral bodies and posterior elements with some degree of malalignment of the spine, the incidence of neurologic deficit is 60%. Ten percent of cases of traumatic cord injury have no evidence of vertebral injury. (These are generally older patients with degenerate spines who have sustained hyperextension injuries.)

In 85% of cases spinal cord injury occurs immediately; 5–10% occur in the immediate post-injury period; 5–10% are late complications.

The single lateral radiograph will miss 15–30% of injuries and the standard three view series will miss between 1% and 10%. CT alone may miss between 8% and 20%. *Note: it is important to note that CT and the standard cervical spine radiographs do not exclude ligamentous instability. Flexion and extension views are required.*

SPECIFIC CERVICAL SPINE INJURIES

C1: the atlas

The Jefferson fracture

This is a comminuted fracture of the ring involving both the anterior and the posterior arches. This causes centripetal displacement of the fractures. Forces are transmitted though the occipital condyles. The aetiology is vertical compression (axial loading), e.g. diving head first into a shallow swimming pool.

Diagnosis:

The open mouth view:

Bilateral offset or spreading of the lateral articular masses of C1 in relation to C2 (**Figs 6.12 and 6.13**).

C2: the axis

Fractures of the dens (odontoid peg) are classified as follows (**Figs 6.14 and 6.15**).

Classification of Odontoid fractures (Anderson and D'Alonzo)

    I: Through the upper peg
   II: Through the base of the peg

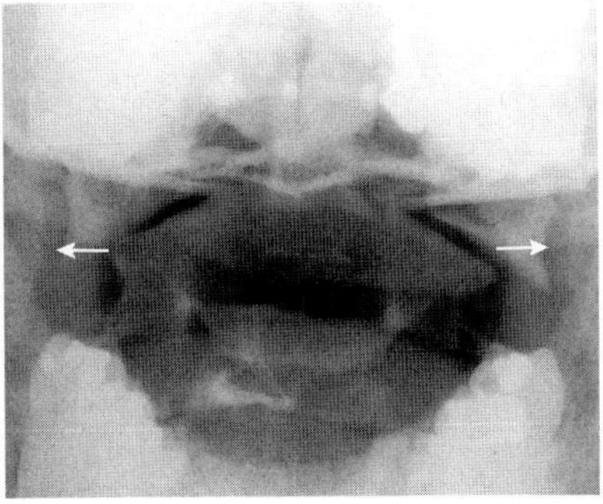

Fig. 6.12 Jefferson fracture, cervical spine peg view. There is lateral displacement of the lateral masses of the atlas, with non-alignment of the lateral masses with the lateral limits of C2.

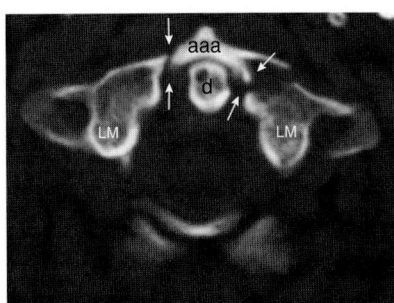

Fig. 6.13 Jefferson fracture (arrows): CT. LM: lateral mass of atlas, d: dens, aaa: anterior arch of atlas.

89

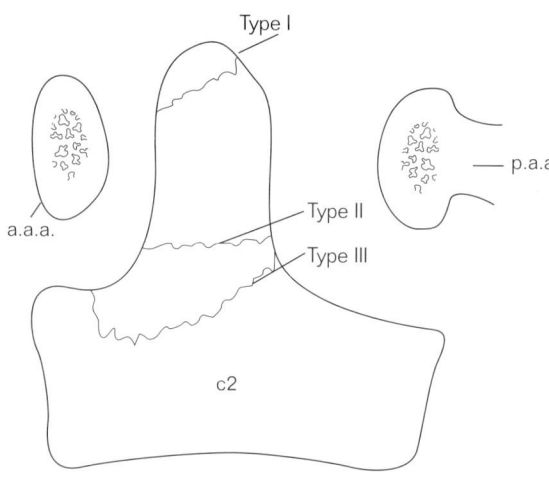

Type I

Type II

Type III

a.a.a.

c2

p.a.a.

Fig. 6.14 Sagittal section through the atlas and the axis demonstrating the classification of peg fractures. a.a.a: anterior arch of atlas, p.a.a: posterior arch of atlas, C2: vertebral body of c2.

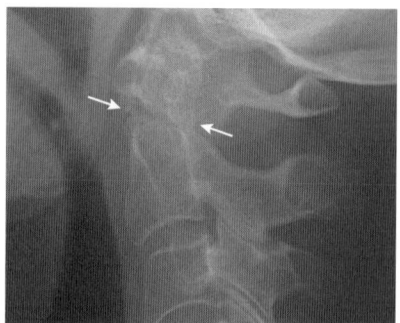

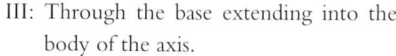

Fig. 6.15 Lateral cervical spine showing peg fracture.

III: Through the base extending into the body of the axis.

The hyperextension teardrop fracture

This is an isolated fracture of the anterior inferior margin of C2. There is an associated tear of the anterior longitudinal ligament (**Figs 6.16 and 6.17**).

The hangman fracture

This is a fracture of the neural arch of C2, and is in effect a traumatic spondylolisthesis of the axis (**Figs. 6.18 and 6.19**).

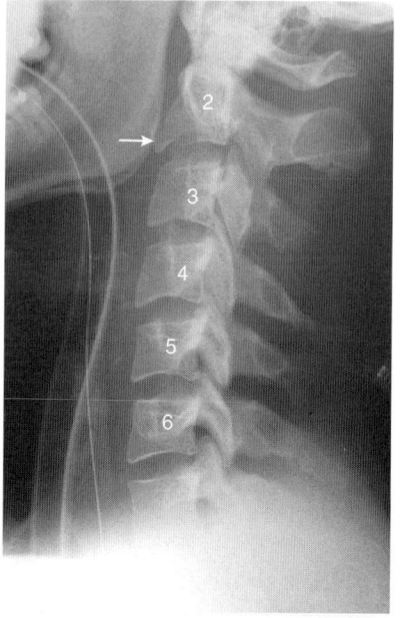

Fig. 6.16 Extension teardrop fracture: neutral position.

Effendi classification for traumatic spondylolisthesis

I. The C2 disc is intact
II. The C2 disc is disrupted
III. There is bilateral facetal dislocation at C2/3 in addition to the pars fracture.

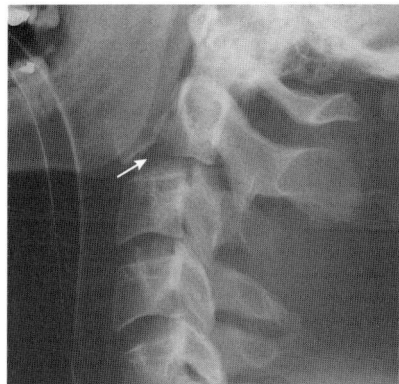

Fig. 6.17 Extension teardrop: hyperextension (same patient as 6.16).

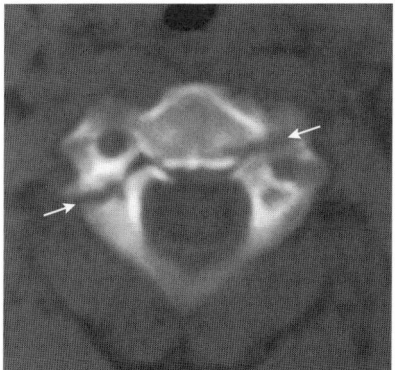

Fig. 6.19 Hangman fracture: CT scan through C2 (same patient as Fig. 6.18) confirming the fracture.

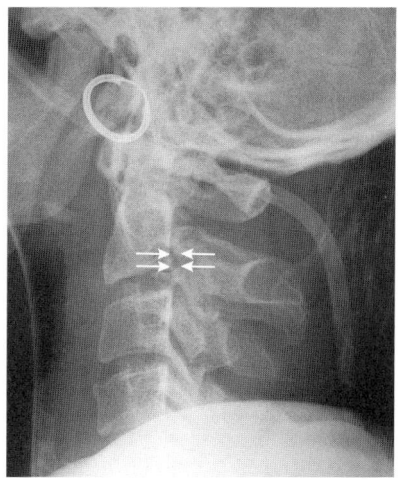

Fig. 6.18 Hangman fracture: lateral cervical spine. There is a fracture (arrows) through the apophysis of C2. (The metallic density is an earring.)

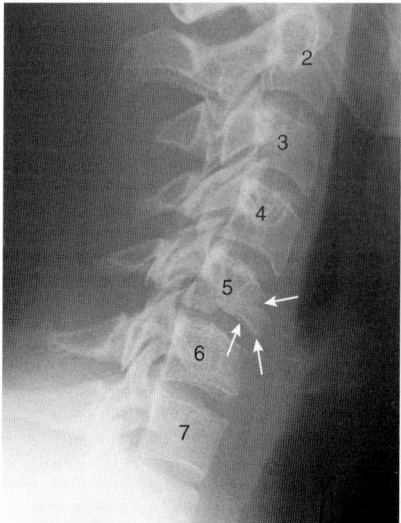

Fig. 6.20 Flexion teardrop fracture: lateral radiograph of cervical spine. There is loss of the normal endplates at the upper and lower borders of C5.

The full force of the injury is transmitted through the apophyseal joints. The weakest part of the neural arch is the interarticular segment of the pedicle. The fracture line extends obliquely, posterosuperior to an anteroinferior location. *Note: an extension teardrop fracture may occur in association with this fracture. If the teardrop fracture is seen, look for the occult hangman fracture. Both are unstable.*

Other vertebral fractures

The flexion teardrop fracture

This is one of the most severe and unstable of injuries (**Fig. 6.20**). It is characterized by

1. Posterior subluxation of the involved vertebra into the spinal canal
2. Fracture of the posterior elements
3. Disruption of the soft tissues including the ligamentum flavum.

Facetal dislocation

The normal orientation of the facets on a lateral cervical spine radiograph is that the superior facet (of the vertebra below) lies anterior to the inferior facet (of the vertebra above). The normal joint space at the facets is 2 mm. In dislocation, the inferior facet is in the anterior position. An intermediate pathology where the facets face each other is called *perched facet*.

The hamburger sign in facetal dislocation

On axial CT, the normal superior and inferior facets with the intervening joint space produce a 'hamburger' appearance, and the facet dislocation gives the appearance of a 'reverse hamburger' (**Fig. 6.21**).

Unilateral facet dislocation

Radiographic features of unifacetal dislocation (**Figs 6.22–6.25**)

1. 30° rotation
2. Apparent loss of the disc space
3. 2–4 mm anterior vertebral displacement
4. Loss of the 'hamburger' at one facet joint.★

(★ denotes CT finding)

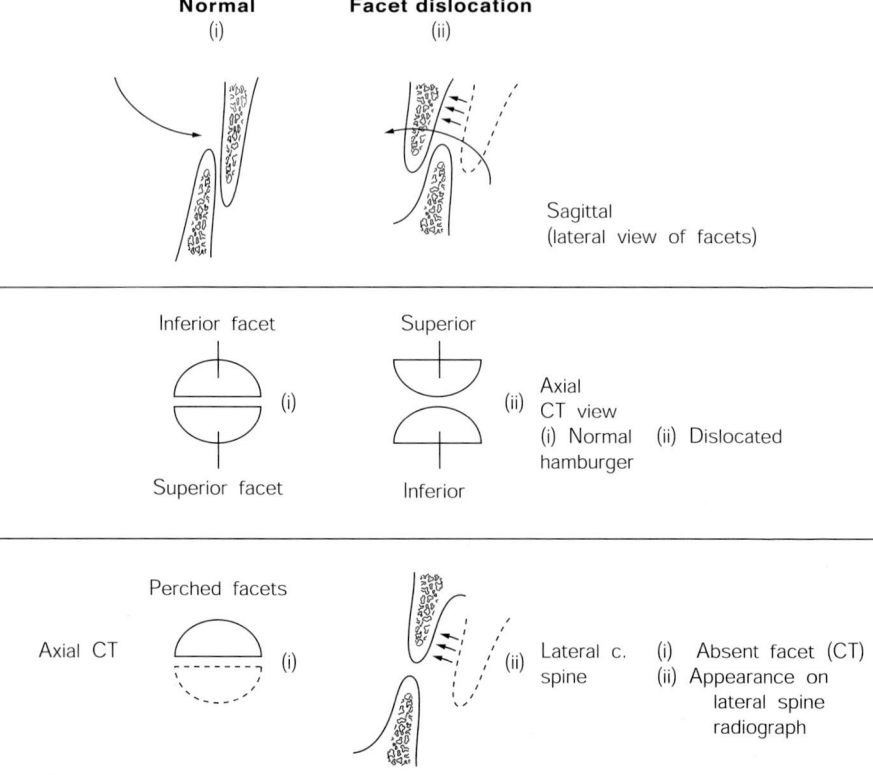

Fig. 6.21 The hamburger sign in facetal dislocation.

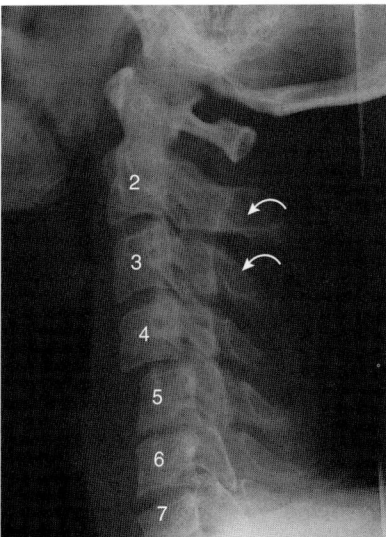

Fig. 6.22 Unifacetal dislocation: lateral cervical spine. There is a facetal dislocation at C4/5. There is anterior subluxation of C4 on C5 and obliquity of the posterior elements above the level of the dislocation (curved arrows).

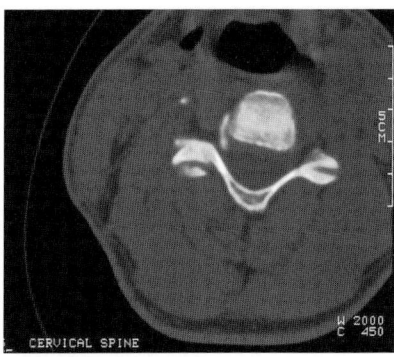

Fig. 6.24 Unifacetal dislocation: axial CT demonstrating the hamburger sign.

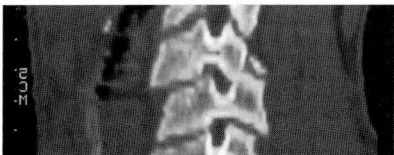

Fig. 6.25 Unifacetal dislocation: CT reconstruction.

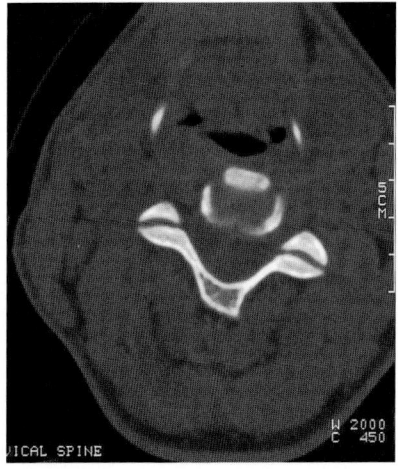

Fig. 6.23 CT demonstrating the normal facetal joints.

Bilateral facet dislocation

Radiological features of bifacetal dislocation (**Fig. 6.26**)

1. No rotation
2. Anterior rotation of 40–50%
3. Loss of the 'hamburger' at the facet joints.*

(* denotes CT finding)

Wedge fracture

This is due to hyperflexion of the cervical spine. There is anterior compression of the vertebral body (**Fig. 6.27**). A disparity of <2 mm between the anterior and the posterior cortex suggests a compression fracture. A disparity of greater than 25% between the height of the anterior and the posterior cortex indicates a

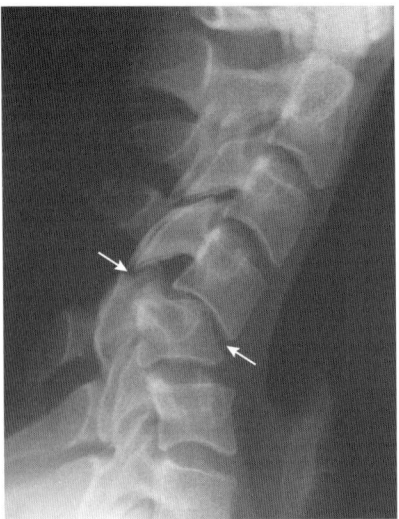

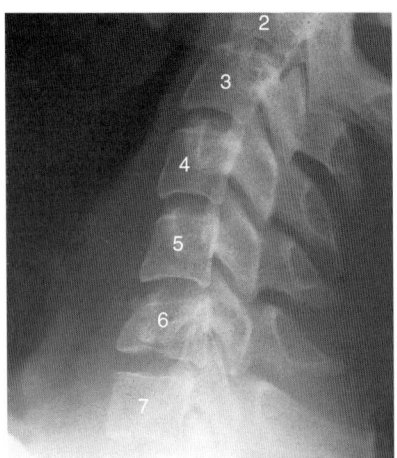

Fig. 6.27 Wedge compression fracture of C6: lateral cervical spine radiograph.

Fig. 6.26 Bifacetal dislocation, lateral cervical spine. There is significant anterior displacement of C4 on C5 (<50%), and disruption of the ligamentous complexes and spinal lines.

tear of the posterior ligamentous complexes, and therefore is a sign of potential instability.

Fractures of the posterior elements: clay-shoveller's fracture

This fracture is due to rotation of the trunk relative to the body. These fractures, if vertical, are stable as the posterior longitudinal ligament remains intact (**Fig. 6.28**) and acts as a splint.

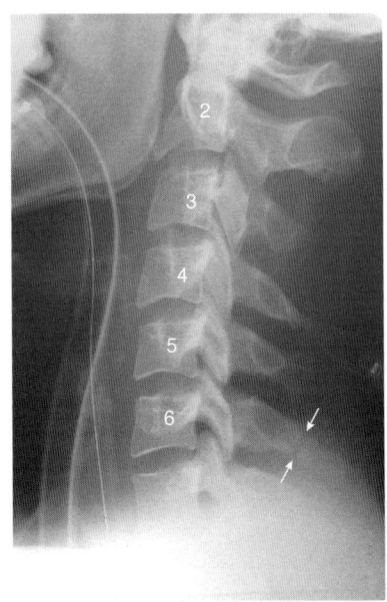

Fig. 6.28 Clay-shoveller's fracture (arrowed).

THORACOLUMBAR INJURIES

Chance fracture

These fractures were originally described in relation to lap belt injuries. They occur at the thoraco-lumbar junction and are often related to significant intraperitoneal visceral injury, notably duodenal rupture and mesenteric tears. In the context of appropriate trauma, finding one should initiate a search for the other.

Classification of Chance fractures (Figs 6.29–6.30)

1. Disruption of the posterior ligaments, articular facets and disc. Spinous process, pedicles and transverse processes intact.

2. Disruption of the posterior elements with extension into the posterior superior or inferior aspect of the vertebral body.

3. Disruption of the posterior elements with an associated transverse fracture of the vertebral body.

Spondylolysis (pars defect)

This is a defect in the pars intraarticularis. Radiologically, this is best demonstrated on the oblique lumbar radiograph as a defect in the 'neck of the Scottie dog' (Fig. 6.31, 6.32a, b).

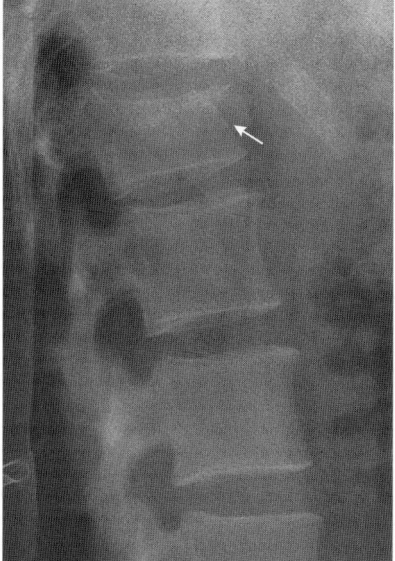

Fig. 6.29 Chance fracture of L1, lateral lumbar spine.

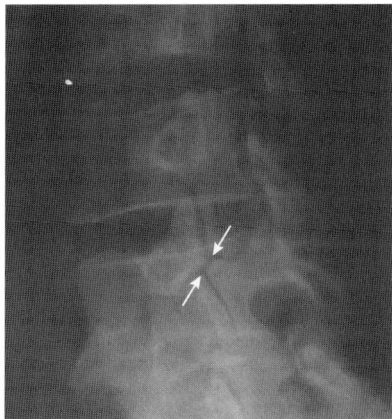

Fig. 6.31 Pars defect; the 'scottie dog' sign. (arrowed).

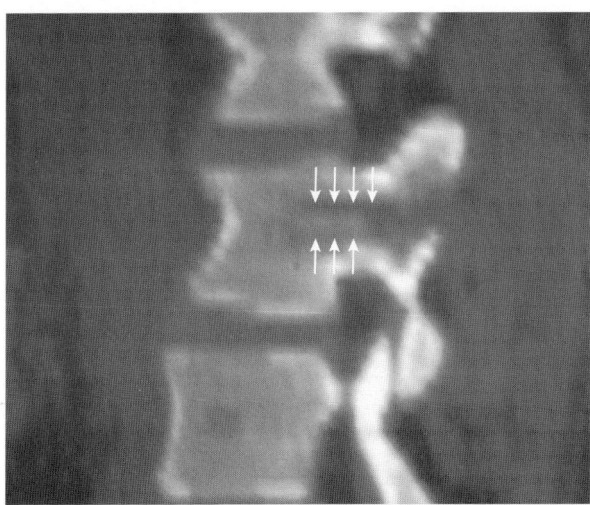

Fig. 6.30 Chance fracture: CT reconstruction showing the extent of the fracture which extends through the posterior elements to, and through, the vertebral body.

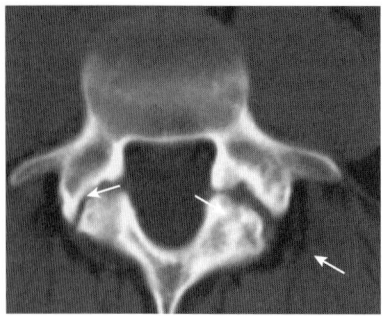

Fig. 6.32a Axial CT, pars defect.

Spondylolisthesis

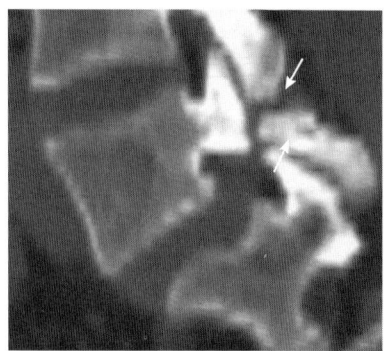

Fig. 6.32b CT reconstruction, pars defect.

This is a bilateral pars defect with anterior displacement of the vertebral body (but not the posterior elements).

DEGENERATIVE DISEASES

Osteoarthritis

Osteoarthritis, or degenerative joint disease (DJD), is the commonest arthritis seen by radiologists. The commonest features of this condition are loss of joint space, reactive sclerosis, osteophytes and subchondral cyst formation (**Fig. 6.33**). Osteoarthritis has been subdivided into two types: primary and secondary. Secondary (i.e. DJD), is the commoner, and is seen in the knees, hips and spine. Primary osteoarthritis is a rarer, familial disease, symmetrically affecting the interphalangeal joints of the hand and the first carpometacarpal joint of the thumb.

Degenerative disc disease (spondylosis)

Degenerative discs may herniate into adjacent neural tissue producing myelopathic or radiculopathic effects with the spinal cord and nerve roots respectively. In addition, the degenerating disc can stimulate osteophyte production which, with ligament hypertrophy and degeneration of the apophyseal vertebral joints, produces a secondary spinal stenosis. Again, this can present as a myelopathy or radiculopathy. Degenerative disc disease occurs most commonly in the lower cervical and lumbar areas (**Figs 6.34 and 6.35**).

Features of degenerative disc disease on the plain radiograph

- Narrowing of the disc space (and, occasionally, gas within the disc)
- Sclerosis of the endplates, and posterior elements
- Osteophytosis.

There is little correlation between patient symptomatology and the radiological changes on plain radiographs of the spine. Cross-sectional techniques, i.e. CT and MRI, elegantly demonstrate disc herniation (**Fig. 6.36**) but it is salutary to

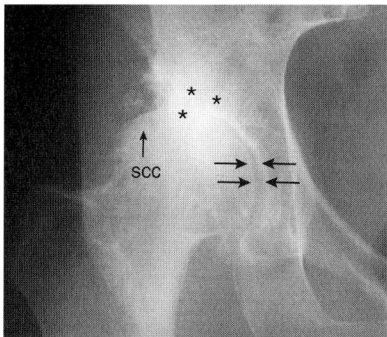

Fig. 6.33 Osteoarthritis of the right hip. Note the loss of joint space (arrows), sclerosis (*) and subchondral cyst (scc).

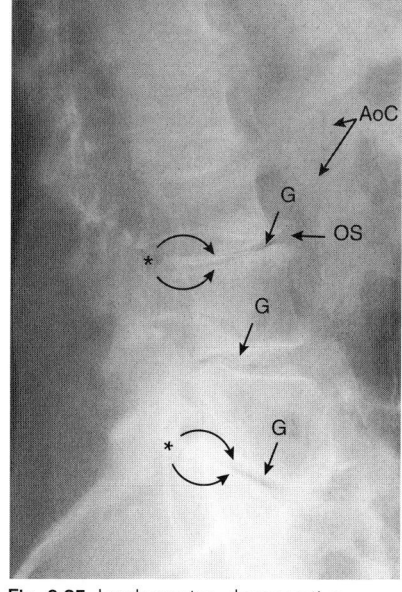

Fig. 6.35 Lumbar spine, degenerative changes. On this lateral view note the loss of alignment, disc space narrowing (*), gaseous degeneration of the disc (G), osteophyte formation (OS) and incidental aortic calcification (AoC)

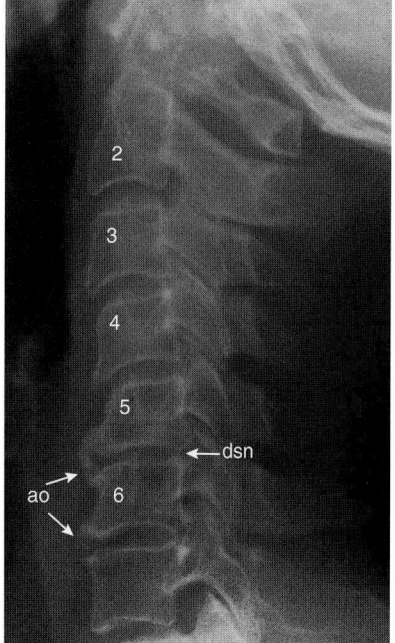

Fig. 6.34 Cervical spine, degenerative changes: lateral cervical spine radiograph. There is disc space narrowing (dsn) at C5/6 and anterior osteophytes (ao) at the lower cervical levels.

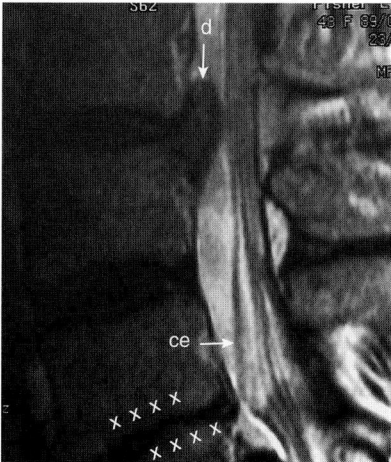

Fig. 6.36 Lumbar disc degeneration and herniation: MRI (T2W sagittal view). d: disc protusion, xx: narrowed disc space, ce: caude equina.

remember that up to 25% of 30-year-old asymptomatic adults have MR evidence of disc protrusions. The protruded disc, therefore, does not necessarily indicate significance.

Paget's disease

Paget's disease is seen both within the spine and the pelvis. The clinical importance is its differentiation from metastatic disease. Paget's disease always begins at a bone end. This is easier to verify in the innominate bone than a vertebral body, but should be sought as an important differentiating point.

Paget's disease of the vertebral body

There is exaggeration and coarsening of the trabecular pattern. This usually leads to enlargement of the vertebral body (**Fig. 6.37**).

Paget's disease of the pelvis

There is coarsening and exaggeration of the bony trabecular pattern and prominence of the iliopectineal line. Check that the changes emanate from the bone end (**Fig. 6.38**).

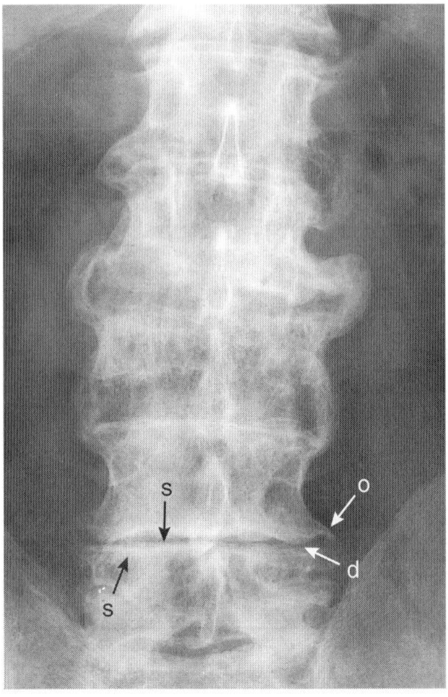

Ankylosing spondylitis

This disease usually presents as an inflammatory arthritis affecting the sacroiliac joints initially, and subsequently the spine. The sacroiliac joint arthropathy consists of cortical erosion, loss of joint space and eventually ankylosis (**Fig. 6.39**). Vertebral involvement generally follows the

Fig. 6.37 Paget's disease of the vertebral body. There is coarsening of the trabecular pattern of L2 and L3 compared to the remaining vertebral bodies. Branching osteophytes are also demonstrated. Note also the concurrent appearances of degenerative disc disease at L4/5 with osteophytes (o), disc space narrowing (d) and sclerosis at the end plates (s).

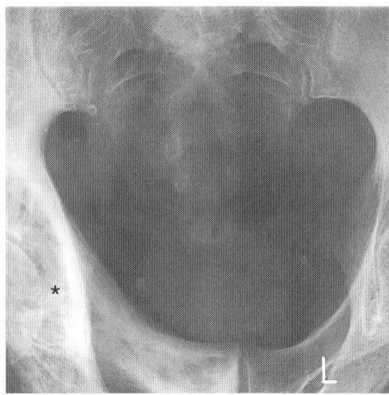

Fig. 6.38 Paget's disease of the pelvis. Note the coarsening of the right innominate bone (*) compared to the left.

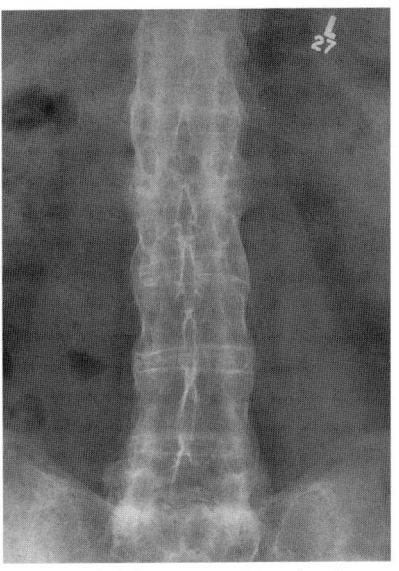

Fig. 6.39 Ankylosing spondylitis: bamboo spine (lumbar spine).

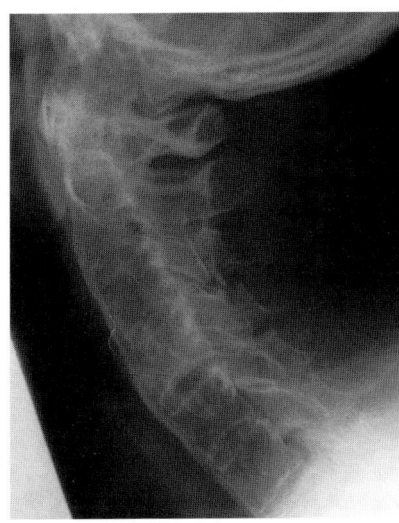

Fig. 6.40 Ankylosing spondylitis: bamboo spine (cervical spine).

sacroiliac disease. The vertebrae become squared, essentially by mineralization of the anterior longitudinal ligament and erosion of the endplate margins. The annulus fibrosis of the discs then ossify on their outer aspects to produce *syndesmophytes*. These syndesmophytes then coalesce to produce the *bamboo spine* (**Fig. 6.40**).

METASTASES

Metastatic bone disease is up to 100 times more frequent than primary bone tumours. Metastases within a vertebra can be lucent (darker than the surrounding bone) or sclerotic (brighter than the surrounding bone). Metastases tend to involve the pedicle of the vertebra (unlike myeloma, which generally involves the vertebral body). On the anterior projection, the pedicles have been likened to two eyes, and the spinous process as a nose. Pedicular infiltration by a lytic tumour therefore, looks like one eye closed or winking at the observer (**Fig. 6.41 and 6.42**).

Tumours that commonly metastasize to bone

- Breast
- Prostate
- Lung
- Lymphoma
- Kidney.

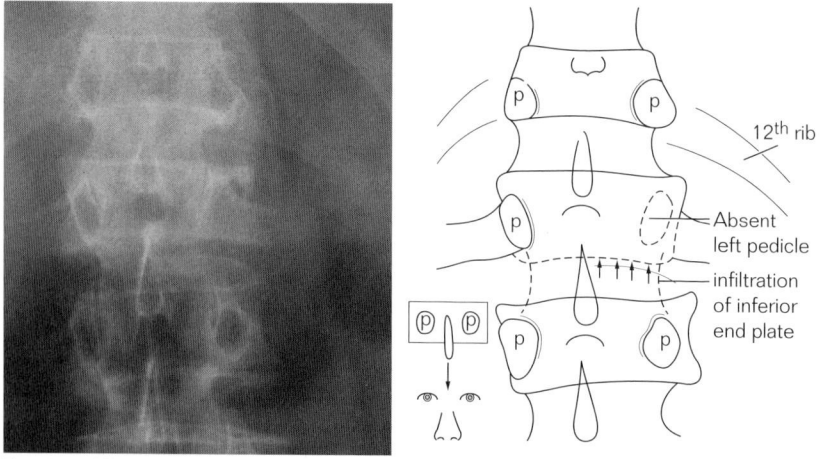

Fig. 6.41 Metastatic disease of the lumbar vertebra (lucent) (absence of the L1 pedicle on the left).

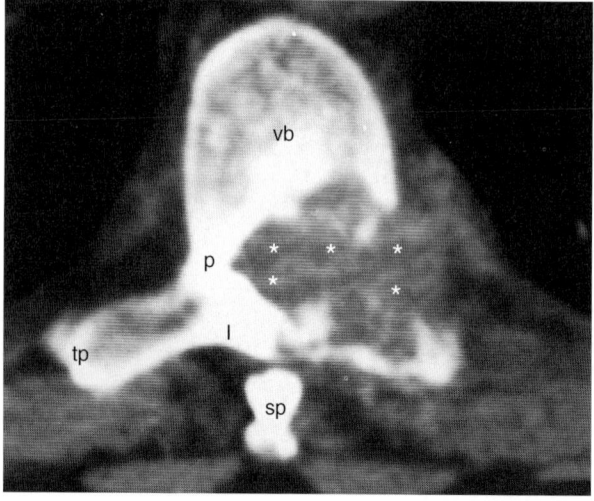

Fig. 6.42 CT metastatic infiltration of the lumbar spine.
vb: vertebral body, p: pedicle, l: lamina, sp: spinous process, tp: transverse process, *: metastatic infiltration.

Two groups of metastases are worthy of further comment: *sclerotic* and *expansile*.

Sclerotic metastases occur with the following malignancies: (**Figs 6.43 and 6.44**)

- Prostate
- Lymphoma
- Breast
- Carcinoid
- Bronchus
- Medulloblastoma.

This can be remembered by the following axiomatic mnemonic: '**P**atchy **L**ong **B**ones **C**an **B**e **M**alignant!'

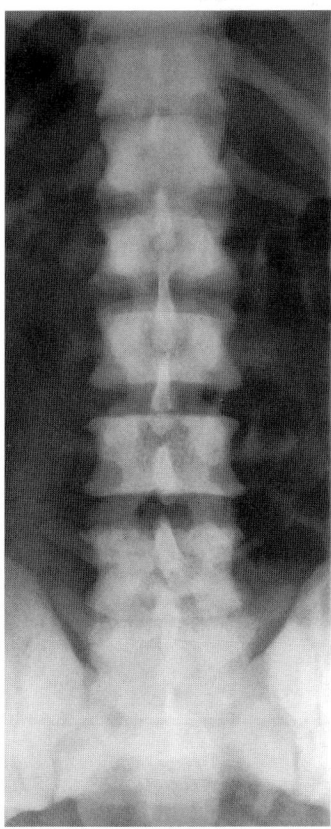

Grossly expansile metastases occur with the following malignancies:

- Melanoma
- Myeloma
- Renal
- Phaeochromocytoma
- Thyroid.

Again, it may be easier to remember these axiomatically: '**M**aggie **M**arches **R**ight **P**ast **T**hem!'

Fig. 6.43 Metastatic disease of the lumbar vertebra (sclerotic). Note the very bright appearance of the vertebral bodies indicating sclerotic infiltration of the vertebral column.

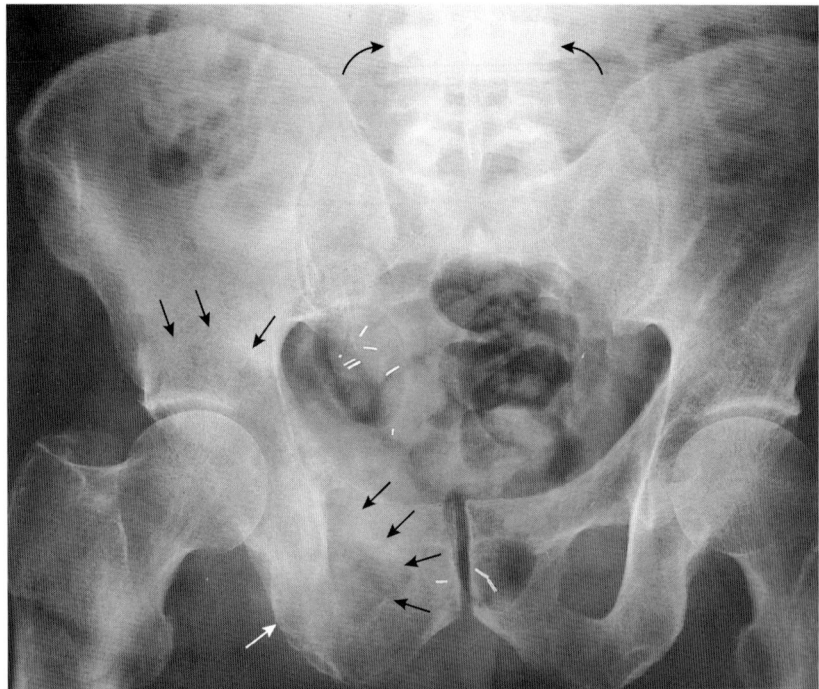

Fig. 6.44 Metastatic disease of the pelvis (sclerotic), involving the right innominate bone (arrows). There is loss of the normal trabecular pattern, compared with the left innominate bone. In addition, the disease does not extend to the bone end and therefore is not Paget's disease. Note also sclerotic infiltration of the L4 vertebral body (curved arrows).

Further Reading

Greenspan A 1992 Orthopaedic radiology: a practical approach. New York: Gower.

Harris J H, Mirvis S 1987 The radiology of acute cervical spine trauma, 2nd edn. Baltimore: Williams & Wilkins.

Helms C A 1995 Fundamentals of skeletal radiology, 2nd edn. Philadelphia: W B Saunders.

7 | Vascular Imaging

Vascular imaging and the techniques of vascular intervention are evolving rapidly. Clinical parameters are constantly being reevalued in the light of new developments. The management of vascular disease represents an area where cooperation between the vascular surgeon and the interventional radiologist is mandatory. Clearly, for reasons of brevity, this short chapter can provide only a brief outline of this developing field. For a fuller description of both vascular and non-vascular interventional techniques the reader is referred to the bibliography at the end of the chapter.

ARTERIAL DISEASES

Aortic aneurysm

The imaging assessment of abdominal (and thoracic) aortic aneurysms is critical in their management paradigm. Initial diagnosis is either by clinical examination and/or ultrasound. The optimal assessment is obtained by spiral CT examination (**Figs 7.1 and 7.2**) and potentially MRI.

Points to note on the CT assessment of an aortic aneurysm:

- Maximum diameter of aneurysm
- Length of infrarenal neck, if present
- Type of aneurysm, e.g. fusiform, saccular
- Appearance of iliac arteries: aneurysmal? diseased?
- Size of kidneys: small may indicate associated renal artery stenosis

- Presence of soft tissue collar around aneurysm to suggest an 'inflammatory' aneurysm
- Presence of important variants such as low left renal vein or circumaortic left renal vein, accessory renal arteries
- Retroperitoneal blood indicating rupture.

Peripheral vascular disease

In the UK, the vascular tree of the lower limb is the most common vascular system to be imaged. However, many other territories can be imaged and assessed, either as a diagnostic test or as a prelude to dedicated intervention.

Transfemoral angiography

Femoral angiography is the gold standard for the evaluation of lower limb peripheral

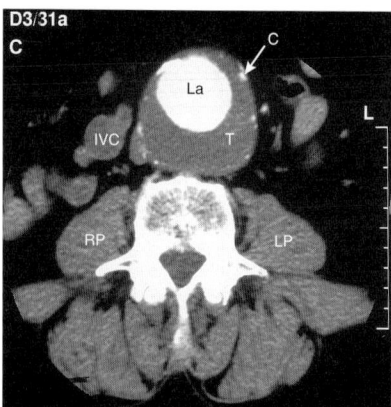

Fig. 7.1 Axial CT slice showing aortic aneurysm. IVC: inferior vena cava, RP: right psoas muscle, LP: left psoas muscle, La: lumen of aortic aneurysm, T: thrombus within aneurysm, C: calcium delineating the endothelium of the aorta.

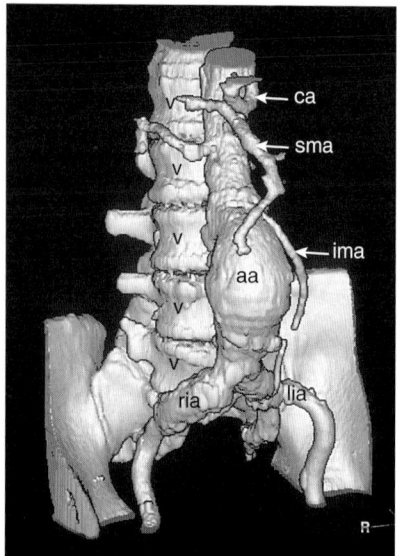

Fig. 7.2 Three-dimensional surface shaded image from spiral CT examination showing abdominal aortic aneurysm. ca: coeliac axis, sma: superior mesenteric artery, ima: inferior mesenteric artery, aa: aortic aneurysm, ria: right common iliac artery, lia: left common iliac artery, v: vertebral column.

vascular disease. This disease is categorized according to the Fontaine classification.

The Fontaine classification

Grade I: no symptoms

Grade IIa: claudication at greater than 200 m

Grade IIb: claudication at less than 200 m

Grade III: rest pain

Grade IV: ulceration and gangrene.

Transfemoral angiography utilizes the modified Seldinger technique, whereby a needle is placed through the anterior wall of the common femoral artery, and a guide wire subsequently passed through the lumen. Once the needle is withdrawn, a pigtail catheter can be 'railroaded' along the wire. The wire is subsequently removed and iodinated contrast injected. Arterial flow pulses the contrast down the lower limb, and images can be recorded using a standard X-ray tube/cassette combination, or a digital camera system (**Figs 7.3 and 7.4**).

Carotid and mesenteric disease

The carotid arteries are best screened by duplex sonography, as there are no associated procedural risks (**Fig. 7.5**; p. 106). Angiography of the carotids should be reserved for those patients with a stong history and evidence of a haemodynamically significant carotid lesion on duplex sonography. Magnetic resonance angiography shows great promise as a diagnostic test for the carotids, and has the advantage (unlike duplex) of not being operator dependent (**Fig. 7.6**; p. 106).

Assessment of mesenteric vessels is performed routinely for occult gastrointestinal bleeding and for suspected 'mesenteric angina', i.e. pain following food ingestion resulting from an inadequate mesenteric

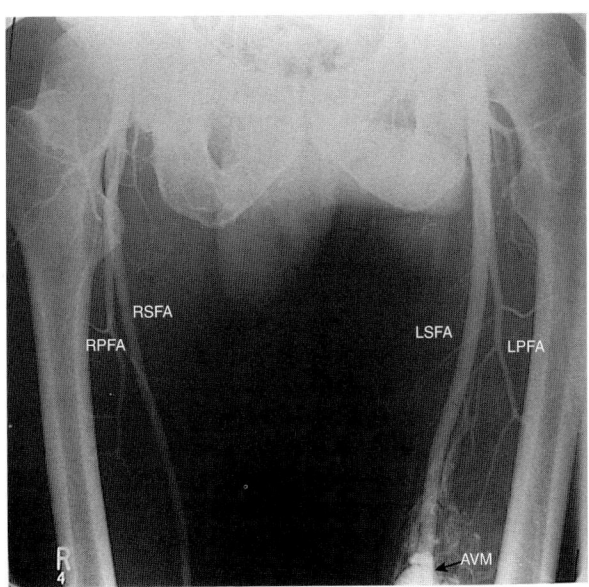

Fig. 7.3 Conventional arteriogram of femoral arteries; note left-sided arteriovenous malformation (AVM). RPFA: right profunda femoris artery, RSFA: right superficial femoral artery, LSFA: left superficial femoral artery, LPFA: left profunda femoris artery.

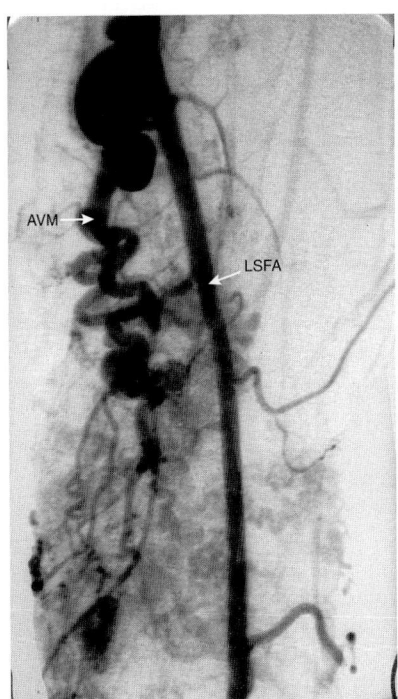

Fig. 7.4 Digital subtraction angiogram of left femoral artery further demonstrating the arteriovenous malformation (AVM). SFA: superior femoral artery.

blood supply. The renal arteries can be imaged in case of hypertension, diminishing renal function and 'flash' pulmonary oedema. Numerous other vascular territories such as the upper limb, bronchial vessels, hepatic and other abdominal vessels and pelvic arteries are imaged for a variety of indications such as trauma, cancer intervention, inflammatory disease, bleeding and suspected occlusive disease. Presently in the UK, most centres continue to rely on diagnostic angiography as the mainstay for the evaluation of these patients.

Percutaneous angioplasty and endovascular stent placement

Angioplasty

Balloon dilatation is the commonest vascular intervention and achieves its effect by fracturing atheromatous plaque and stretching the tunica media. Gruntzig and Hopff described the first reliable angioplasty balloon catheter in 1974.

105

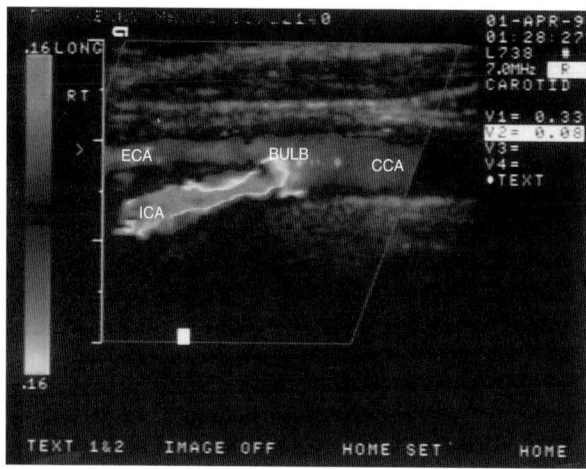

Fig. 7.5 Colour Doppler examination of carotid bifurcation. CCA: common carotid artery, ECA: external carotid artery, ICA: internal carotid artery.

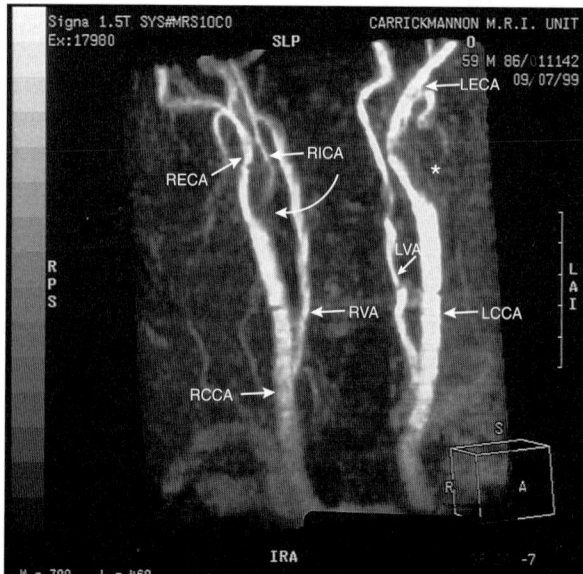

Fig. 7.6 Magnetic resonance angiogram (MRA) of carotid and vertebral arteries in the neck using two-dimensional time-of-flight (tof) imaging. Note the stenosis (curved arrow) of the proximal right internal carotid artery (RICA) and the occlusion of the left internal carotid artery(*). RECA/LECA: right/left external carotid artery, RCCA/LCCA: right/left common carotid artery, RVA/LVA: right/left vertebral artery.

Indications for lower limb angioplasty

1. Intermittent claudication of 200 m or less (Fontaine IIb)
2. Rest pain (Fontaine III)
3. Gangrene or ulceration (Fontaine IV)
4. A stenosis that compromises graft patency.

Contraindications to angioplasty

Absolute

1. Recent arterial thrombosis

Relative

1. Bleeding diathesis
2. Long iliac occlusions: primary stent placement preferred

3. Total aortic occlusions: stenting again is an option
4. Aneurysm adjacent to stenosis.

Angioplasty technique

Access is obtained via the most appropriate vessel and a wire is persuaded across the stenosis/occlusion. A balloon catheter is then passed along the wire and sited appropriately using radiopaque markers. The balloon is inflated using an inflation device and on completion a check arteriogram is performed to ensure a good result and rule out potential complications. Pressure measurements can be taken across the lesion to ensure there is no significant residual pressure gradient (**Figs 7.7 and 7.8**). Anticoagulant and antispasmodic therapy may be necessary during the procedure.

Risks of angioplasty:

* Hospital mortality: 0.07–0.4%
* Limb loss: 0.4%
* Complications at the puncture site: thrombosis, haematoma, pseudoaneurysm, arteriovenous fistula
* Complications at the angioplasty site: thrombosis, perforation, rupture, spasm.

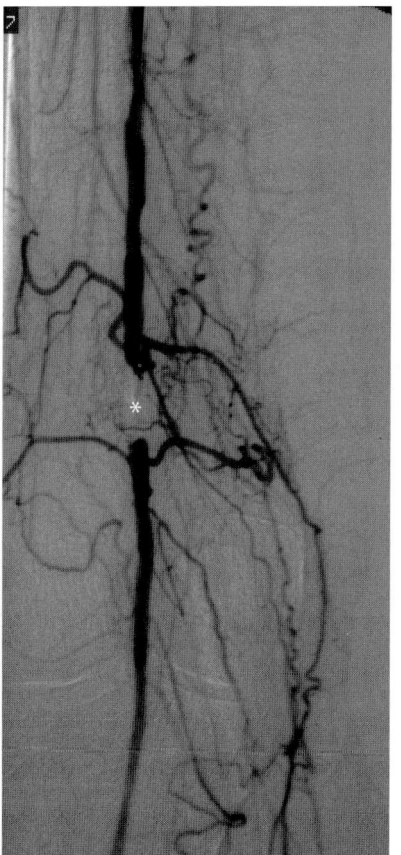

Fig. 7.7 Angioplasty, short popliteal occlusion(∗).

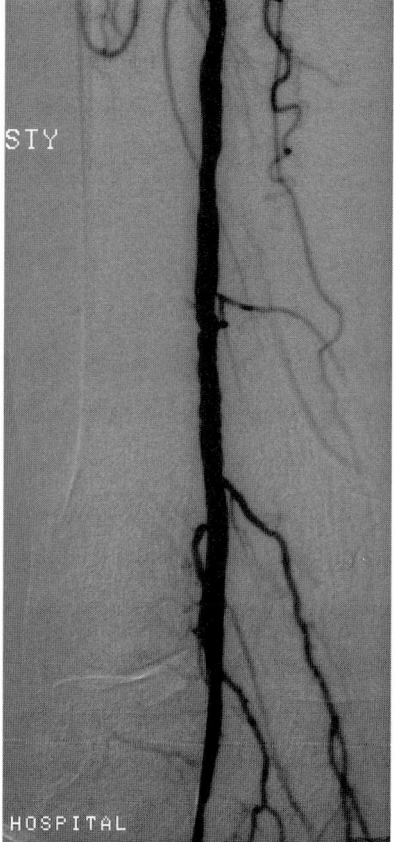

Fig. 7.8 Angioplasty, post-5 mm balloon dilatation. Vessel recannulized.

Long-term results of angioplasty

In general terms the larger the vessel, the better the patency. For example, the 2-year patency of iliac angioplasty is 80–90%, whereas in the popliteal artery it is approximately 50%. A short stenosis with good inflow and run-off vessels is more likely to have a successful outcome than a long stenosis with poor inflow and outflow vessels.

Other vascular territories that may benefit from angioplasty

- Lower limb: iliac, femoral, popliteal, tibial
- Upper limb: subclavian, brachial
- Head and neck: carotid, vertebral
- Body: aorta, renal, mesenteric.

Endovascular stent placement

A large number of stents are available for use in the vascular system. They are made of a variety of materials but in general terms can be described as self-expanding or balloon-expanding.

Indication for placement of stents

- Failed angioplasty: reocclusion, elastic recoil, residual stenosis (**Figs 7.9 and 7.10**), dissection
- Renal ostial stenosis
- Complete iliac and aortic occlusions.

Vascular stents normally have large gaps in the interstices of their metallic framework. For specific pathologies, covered stents may be utilized.

Indications for covered stent placement

- Arteriovenous fistula
- Vascular trauma (penetrating, e.g. bullet)
- Arterial rupture due to angioplasty
- Exclusion of aneurysm, especially aortic and iliac (**Figs 7.11 and 7.12**).

Thrombolysis

Thrombolysis is enzymatic or accelerated thromboembolism dissolution to facilitate

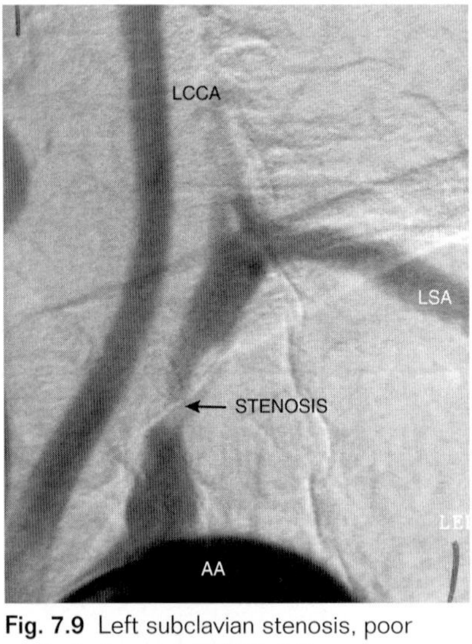

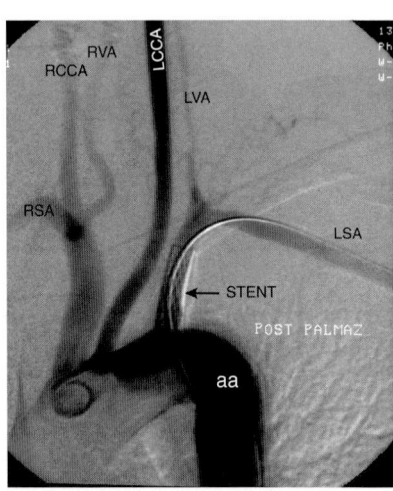

Fig. 7.9 Left subclavian stenosis, poor angioplasty result. LCCA: left common carotid artery, LSA: left subclavian artery, AA: aortic arch.

Fig. 7.10 Appearances post-stent placement. RSA/LSA: right/left subclavian artery, RCCA/LCCA: right/left common carotid artery, RVA/LVA: right/left vertebral artery, aa: aortic arch.

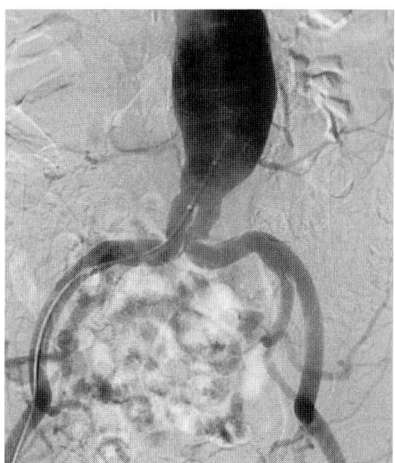

Fig. 7.11 Abdominal aortic aneurysm: digital subtraction angiogram.

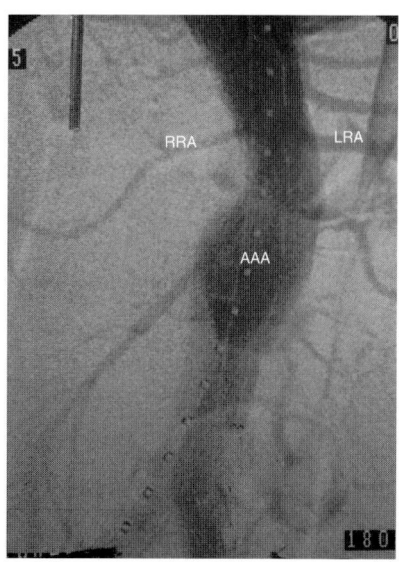

Fig. 7.12 Exclusion of aneurysm following bifurcated aortic stent graft placement. RRA/LRA: right/left renal artery, AAA: aortic aneurysm sac.

vascular patency. There are essentially three agents in common usage: streptokinase, tissue plasminogen activator and urokinase.

Steptokinase (SK) is derived from the group C, β-haemolytic streptococcus. It has the longest half-life of the three. It has a high affinity for plasminogen, therefore requiring adjunctive heparinization, and also has the side-effect of producing systemic lysis. Its biological half-life is 23 minutes, and is administered at a rate of 5000–10 000 u/h.

Tissue plasminogen activator (tPA) was originally produced from vascular human uterine endothelial cells, until manufactured using recombinant DNA technology (rtPA). It has a lower affinity for plasminogen than SK and therefore produces less systemic lytic effect. Its biological half-life is 5 minutes, and its administration rate is 0.5–1.0 mg/h.

Urokinase (UK) was originally isolated from human fetal kidney. Again, this is less likely to produce a systemic lytic state than SK, but can produce self-limiting rigors. Its biological half-life is 12–16 minutes, and administration rate is around 50 000 u/h.

Thrombolytic therapy is administered through a catheter inserted percutaneously and placed directly within the thrombus, and is administered using an infusion pump. Dosage regimens vary, but in essence, there are low-dose infusion techniques, which require longer treatment times but may be safer, and there are higher dose accelerated techniques such as *pulse spray* which can achieve a more rapid clinical response.

Indications for thrombolysis (lower limb ischaemia)
- Occluded grafts
- Distal arterial thrombosis extending into the trifurcation vessels
- Distal arterial embolus extending into the trifurcation vessels
- Proximal thrombosis with poor run-off (**Figs 7.13 and 7.14**).

Indications for vascular surgery
- Failure of thrombolysis
- Contraindication to thrombolysis

- Neurological signs (sensory or motor) at time of presentation
- Proximal, i.e. aortoiliac thrombosis
- Ischaemia for more than 14 days.

Note: If the disease is proximal and there are neurological signs, consider surgery first. If the disease is distal, and there are no neurological signs, consider thrombolysis first.

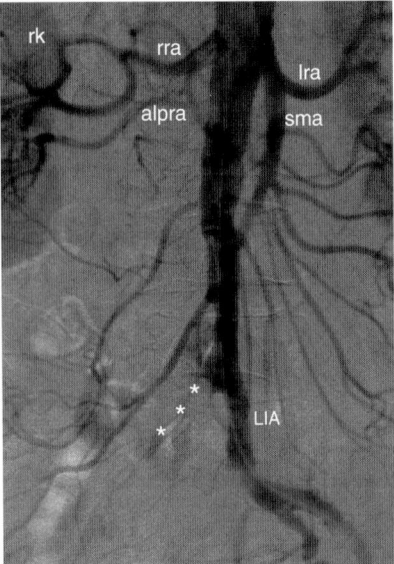

Fig. 7.13 Proximal thrombosis with poor run-off. *** Course of the right iliac artery, rk: right kidney, rra/lra: right/left renal artery, sma: superior mesenteric artery, alpra: accessory lower polar renal artery. LIA: left iliac artery.

Contraindications to thrombolysis:

Absolute

- Active bleeding
- Intracranial tumour
- Stroke <6 months; transient ischaemic attack <2 months.

Relative

- Bleeding diathesis
- Hypertension
- Hepatorenal failure
- Recent abdominal surgery <10 days
- Recent trauma <10 days
- Potential bleeding site: peptic ulcer, postpartum uterus, diabetic retinopathy.

Informed consent with thrombolysis

Practice will vary, but the following points are recommended as those which should be discussed with the patient and should

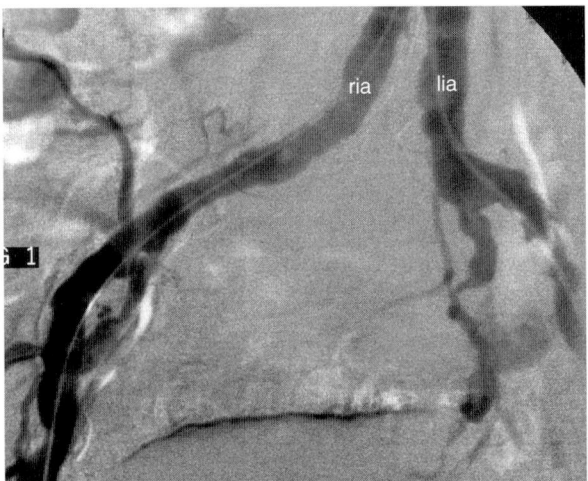

Fig. 7.14 Lower limb vessels following thrombolysis and completion angioplasty. ria/lia: right/left iliac artery. (Same patient as Fig. 7.13).

be documented in the notes as having being discussed with the patient

- The risk of stroke is 2%
- The risk of bleeding requiring treatment is 5% (not requiring treatment, 15%)
- The limb salvage rate with thrombolysis is 75%
- Surgery may be required if there is treatment failure or complication
- Lysis may require 24 hours or longer to complete
- Lysis is often painful, and parenteral analgesia may be given for the duration of treatment.

Arterial embolization

The deliberate occlusion of vessels using various embolic materials requires an intricate knowledge of vascular anatomy and variants thereof. These procedures are highly technically demanding, require high-quality imaging and, sometimes, considerable time and patience.

Commonly used embolic agents

- Absorbable gelatin sponge
- Polyvinyl alcohol particles
- Metallic coils
- Alcohol (95–99%)
- Isobutyl-2-cyanoacrylate (glue).

Indications for percutaneous arterial embolization

- Active bleeding
  (a) gastrointestinal (mesenteric)
  (b) haemoptysis (bronchial)
  (c) trauma – especially pelvic, renal, hepatic and splenic arteries (**Figs 7.15 and 7.16**)
- Tumour palliation
  (a) liver metastases, for neuroendocrine tumours, hepatoma
  (b) other tumours such as hypervascular metastases, and renal cell carcinoma prior to surgery
- Uterine fibroids.

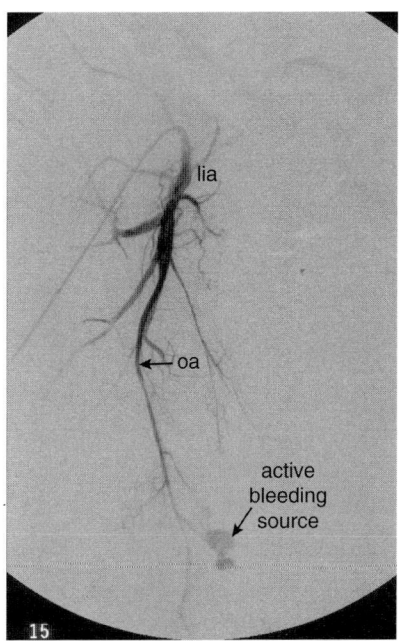

Fig. 7.15 Active bleeding from obturator artery (oa) in patient with pelvic fractures. lia: left iliac artery.

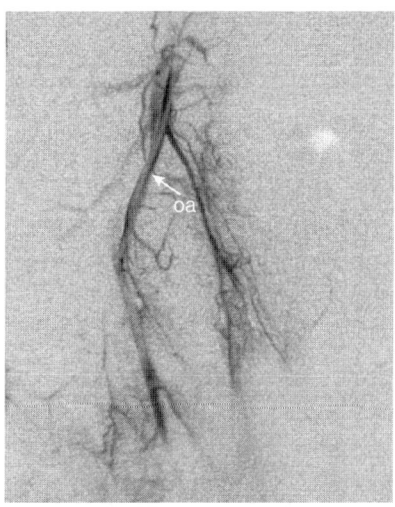

Fig. 7.16 Post-embolization of obturator artery (oa) with gel foam, no further bleeding.

111

VENOUS DISEASES

Current methods of evaluation

There are two commonly utilized methods of evaluating the veins of the lower limb:

- Ascending phlebography (the *venogram*)
- Ultrasound/Doppler venography.

Venography has been the gold standard in examining deep vein patency until recently (**Fig. 7.17**). Its main disadvantages are:

- Venography requires ionizing radiation
- The procedure involves cannulation of a foot vein
- The injected IV contrast carries a small risk of morbidity and mortality.

A deep venous thrombosis produces the classical 'tramline' appearance (**Fig. 7.18**).

Duplex colour Doppler sonography

Colour Doppler sonography utilizes the Doppler effect. This effect detects a change caused by red blood cell movement. The received information can be made audible, or visible, either as a spectral wave, or a colour. The combination of this colour and a real-time image is called *duplex* (**Fig. 7.19**). All three displayed simultaneously (colour + spectrum + real-time image) is called *triplex* (**Fig. 7.20;** p. 114).

Sonographic evaluation of deep venous thrombosis

Ultrasound allows direct visualization of the lower limb veins. The examination begins with a transverse scan through the groin at the level of the femoral vessels. Some authors have likened the configuration of these three vessels to the appearance of Mickey Mouse (**Fig. 7.21;** p. 114).

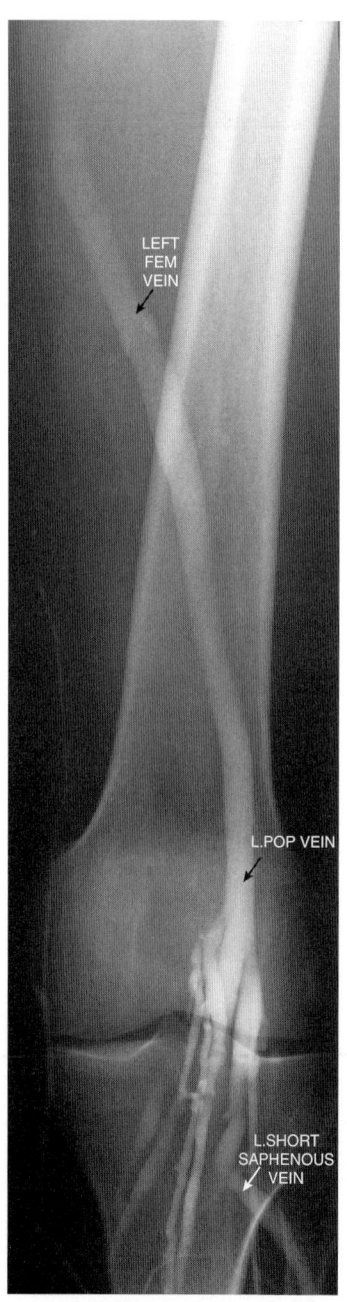

LEFT FEM VEIN

L.POP VEIN

L.SHORT SAPHENOUS VEIN

Fig. 7.17 Ascending venogram demonstrating the normal popliteal and femoral veins.

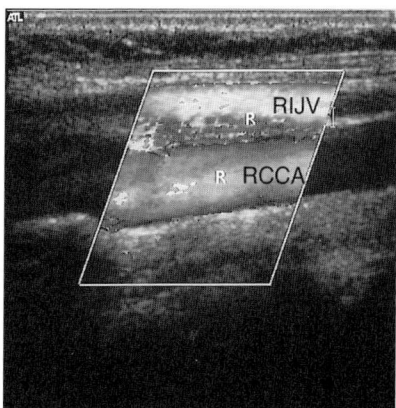

Fig. 7.19 Ultrasound duplex image. RIJV: right internal jugular vein, RCCA: right common carotid artery.

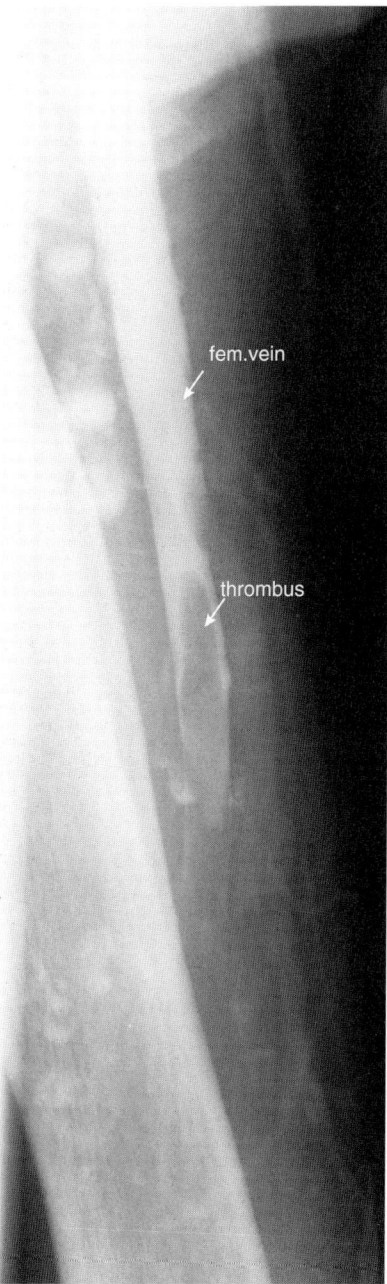

Fig. 7.18 Ascending venogram demonstrating thrombus in the femoral vein.

The normal common femoral and long saphenous veins should be completely

compressible with light pressure from the ultrasound probe. The adjoining artery should not be compressible. Failure to achieve this venous compressibility is strongly suspicious of thrombus (**Figs 7.22–7.24**).

Most authors suggest that compressibility should be tested, as described, at the femoral and popliteal levels. In addition, transverse images may be performed at 1-cm levels between the groin and knee to confirm compressibility.

Phasic flow

Normally there is a phasicity observed within the veins during the respiratory cycle (**Figs 7.25 and 7.26;** p. 115). By stopping respiration and performing a *valsalva manoeuvre* (e.g. ask the patient to 'bear down' as in simulated defecation), the venous flow, monitored at the groin, should stop. This indicates patency more cranially, i.e. at the iliac and caval levels (**Figs 7.27 and 7.28;** p. 116–117).

Similarly, by squeezing the calf muscles, a jet of blood can be detected normally, at groin level. This manoeuvre, the *calf squeeze*, confirms venous patency at

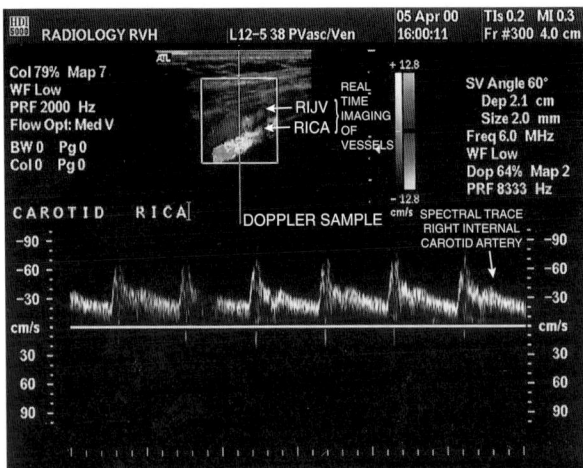

Fig. 7.20 Ultrasound triplex image. RIJV: right internal jugular vein, RICA: right internal carotid artery.

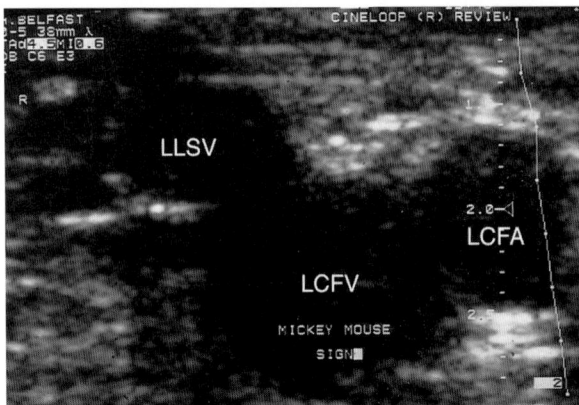

Fig. 7.21 Transverse image through the femoral vessels. The 'Mickey Mouse' sign. LLSV: left long saphenous vein, LCFA: left common femoral artery, LCFV: left common femoral vein.

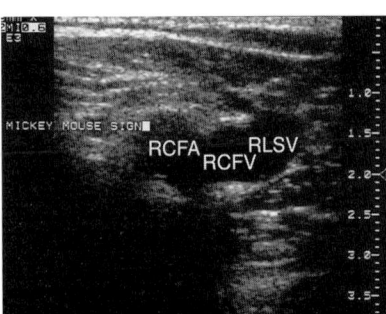

Fig. 7.22 Transverse section through groin. Normal appearances. RCFA: right common femoral artery, RCFV: right common femoral vein, RLSV: right long saphenous vein.

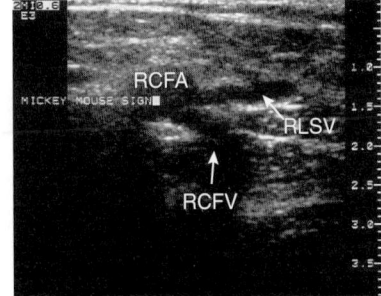

Fig. 7.23 Transverse section following compression. Normal appearances. RCFA: right common femoral artery, RCFV: right common femoral vein, RLSV: right long saphenous vein.

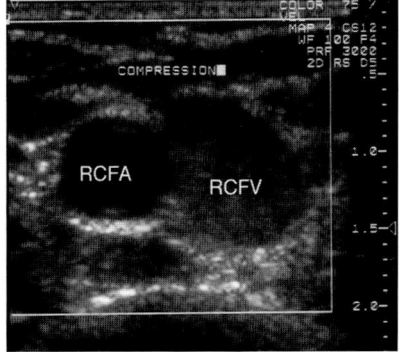

Fig. 7.24 Transverse section with compression. Femoral thrombosis. Note the enlarged and echogenic right common femoral vein which fails to compress (RCFV). RCFA: right common femoral artery.

a lower level (**Fig. 7.29**). A duplex examination of the leg should, with experience, be achievable within 15 minutes. Duplex has a sensitivity of 98% at femoral and popliteal level for clot detection.

Pulmonary embolism

Pulmonary embolism is underdiagnosed, and failure to recognize and treat this condition can have disastrous consequences for the patient.

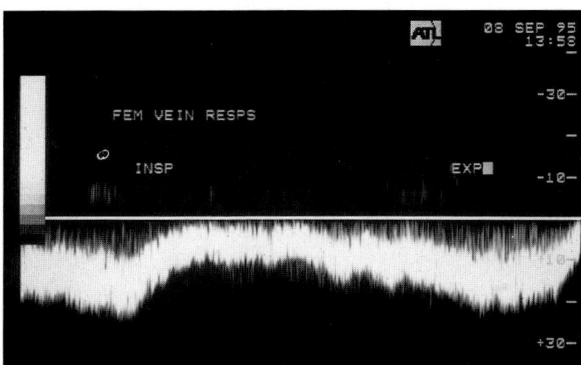

Fig. 7.25 Doppler spectrum: normal phasicity.

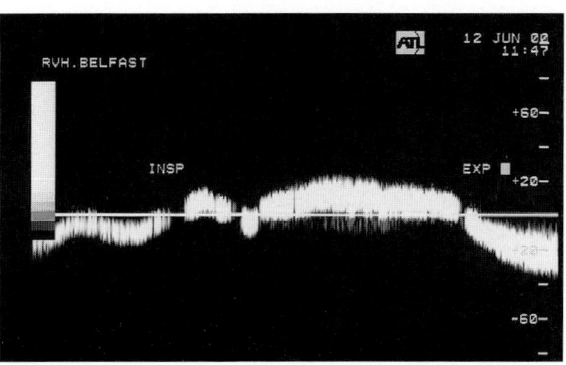

Fig. 7.26 Doppler spectrum: effect of arrested respiration.

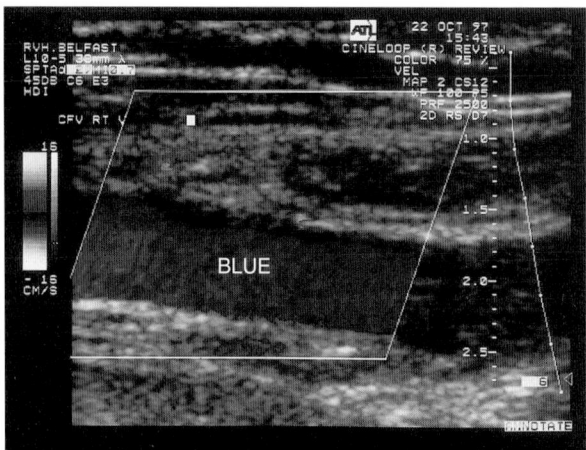

Fig. 7.27 Normal venous colour flow.

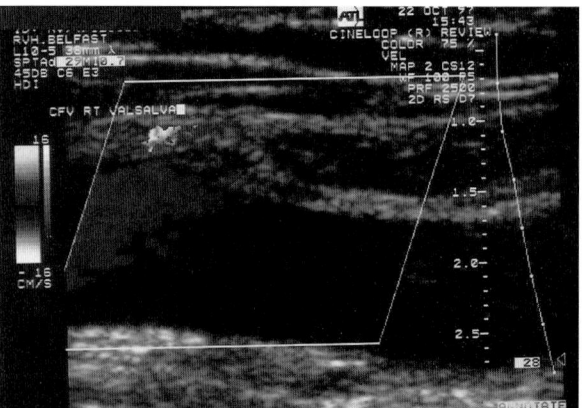

Fig. 7.28 Arrested flow in the femoral vein following valsalva manoeuvre.

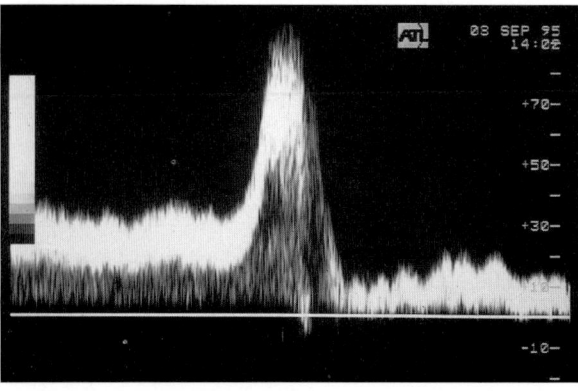

Fig. 7.29 Doppler spectrum: the calf squeeze.

Imaging of pulmonary embolus

- Chest x-ray (frequently normal).
- Ventilation/perfusion scan. Almost 100% reliability when described as normal. The finding of a clear mismatch (i.e. a ventilated but non-perfused region) indicates a high probability of pulmonary embolus.
- Spiral CT angiography (increasingly accepted as frontline investigation).
- MRA (may develop as a major additional investigation).
- Pulmonary angiography (probably still the gold standard; **Fig. 7.30**).

Pulmonary angiography is performed usually with a femoral venous approach. A catheter is persuaded into the right atrium and through the tricuspid valve into the right ventricle and subsequently the pulmonary arteries. Imaging of both lungs is performed selectively and pressure measurements may be taken. If a large quantity of thrombus is present proximally (**Fig. 7.30**), this may be disrupted

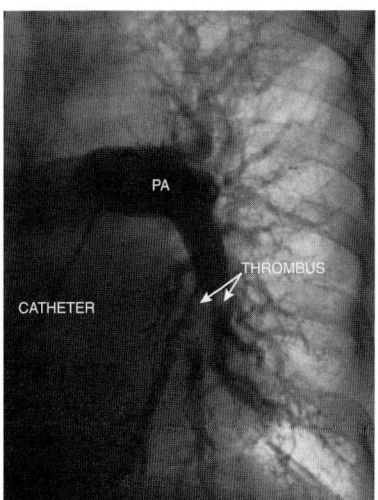

Fig. 7.30 Left pulmonary arteriogram with thrombus seen in the descending pulmonary artery (PA).

mechanically and/or be infused with thrombolytic agent via the catheter.

Venous intervention

Vena caval filters

Inferior vena caval filters are placed to prevent the passage of thrombus from the lower limbs and pelvis to the pulmonary circulation. Following pulmonary embolism the risk of dying from recurrence is 30% if untreated. Despite adequate anticoagulation, 18% may have recurrent emboli.

Filters are classified as:

- Permanent
- Temporary: these are modified catheters and some component remains outside the body. The efficiency of these devices is unproven at present.

Indications for filter placement

Definite

- Proven pulmonary embolus while receiving anticoagulation therapy
- Pulmonary embolus with a contraindication to anticoagulant therapy
- Complications of anticoagulant therapy requiring discontinuation

Controversial

- Thrombus in iliac/femoral veins
- Prolonged immobilization, trauma patients
- Orthopaedic surgery with history of previous DVT.

Indications for temporary filter placement

- Lower limb venous thrombolysis
- Prophylaxis required for short period of time, e.g. surgery
- Pregnant women with deep venous thrombosis.

Inferior vena caval filters are inserted via the femoral, jugular or brachial vein using a percutaneous approach. A cavogram is obtained to delineate the level of the renal veins and to confirm absence of clot in the IVC (**Fig. 7.31**). The filter is then released from a constrained delivery system usually below the level of the renal veins (**Fig. 7.32**). Occasionally it is necessary to place the filter above the level of the renal veins.

Indications for suprarenal filter placement

- Pregnancy: infrarenal filters may be compressed by the enlarging uterus
- Gonadal or renal vein thrombus
- Thrombus extending above the renal veins.

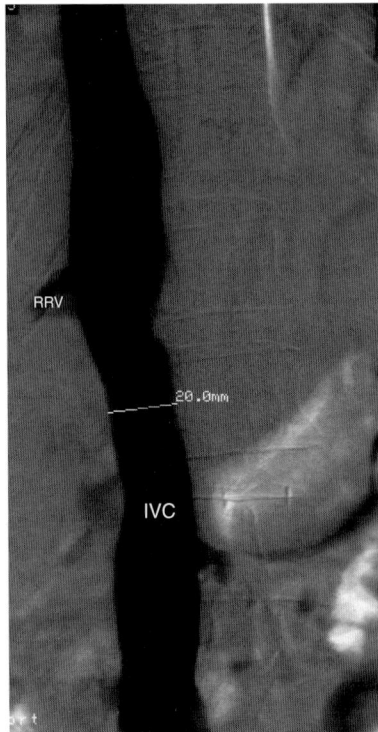

Fig. 7.31 Cavogram showing no thrombus within IVC. RRV: right renal vein, IVC: inferior vena cava.

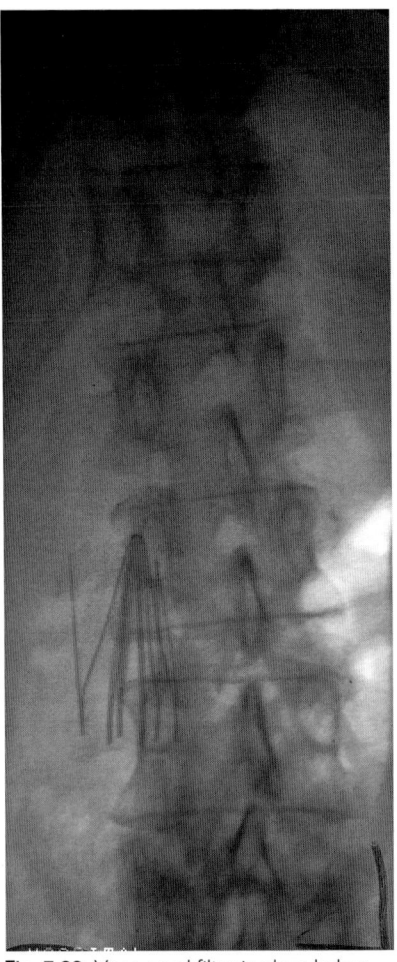

Fig. 7.32 Vena caval filter in place below the level of the renal veins.

Complications of inferior vena caval filter placement:

- Femoral vein thrombosis
- Bleeding at the puncture site
- Caval thrombosis (10%) (most asymptomatic)
- Recurrent embolus (2%)
- Filter migration
- Vena cava perforation and pericaval fibrosis.

Venous angioplasty

Venous angioplasty is normally performed for benign narrowing of veins resulting in venous obstruction. The technique is similar to arterial angioplasty except that venous stenoses are often extremely tight and long inflation times with high pressure balloons are sometimes required. Venous stenoses related to haemodialysis patients are the most frequent indication (**Figs 7.33 and 7.34**).

Venous stenting

Venous stenting is most often performed for malignant conditions particularly superior vena caval obstruction (SVCO).

Causes of malignant SCVO

1. Bronchogenic carcinoma
2. Lymphoma
3. Mediastinal metastatic deposits
4. Mesothelioma.

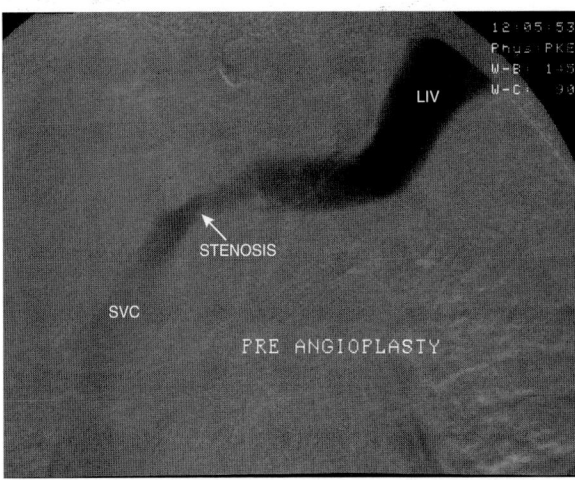

Fig. 7.33 Innominate vein stenosis in a dialysis patient. LIV: left innominate vein, SVC: superior vena cava.

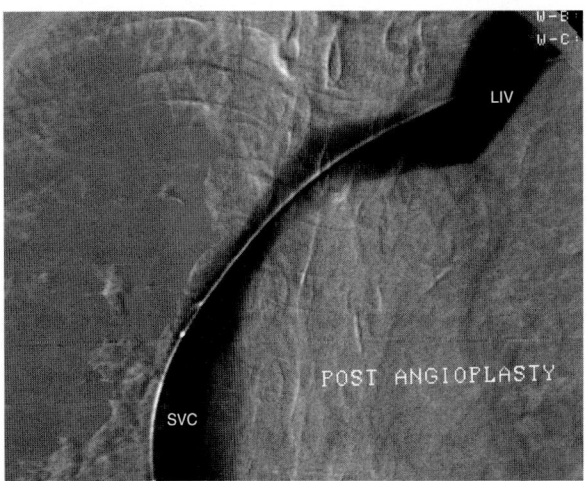

Fig. 7.34 Angiographic result following 12 mm balloon dilatation. LIV: left innominate vein, SVC: superior vena cava.

Increasingly stenting is becoming the first-line treatment for malignant SVCO; however, it should be remembered that lymphoma and small cell carcinoma may show a good early response to radiotherapy.

A tissue diagnosis is clearly indicated before deciding on therapy. The IVC may also be stented in malignant disease (**Figs 7.35 and 7.36**).

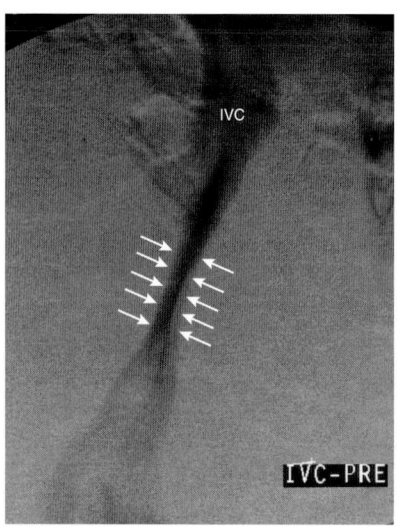

Fig. 7.35 Inferior vena caval stenosis due to adrenal carcinoma (arrows).

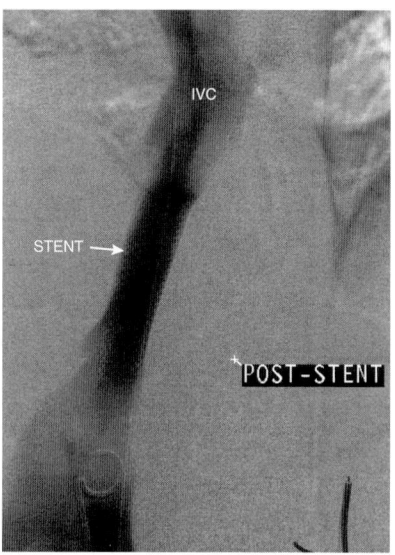

Fig. 7.36 Improvement of stenosis following stent placement.

Further Reading

Belli A M 1994 Practical interventional radiology of the peripheral vascular system. London: Edward Arnold.

Ellis P K, Boyd C S 1999 Interventional radiology for the surgeon. Association of Surgeons in Training Yearbook 1998/1999. London: Rowan Group.

Merritt C R B 1992 Doppler color imaging. New York: Churchill Livingstone.

Watkinson A, Adam A 1996 Interventional radiology – a practical guide, 1st edn. Oxford: Radcliffe Medical Press.

Wojtowycz M 1995 Handbook of interventional radiology and angiography, 2nd edn. St Louis: Mosby.

Index

Page numbers in italics refer to figures and tables